The Hospice of St Francis
A Place and Time

Julian Ashbourn

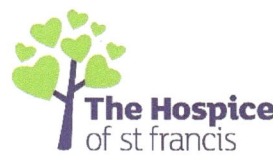

Copyright © 2017 The Hospice of St Francis

All rights reserved.

ISBN 10: 1544693230

ISBN 13: 978-1544693231

Dedication

This book is dedicated to the large number of doctors, nurses, administrative staff and volunteers who together transform the Hospice from a clinical building complex into a wonderful entity of care which illuminates the lives of all those who come into contact with it. While this may be true of many such establishments, The Hospice of St Francis is uniquely blessed in this regard and this uniqueness comes entirely from the people involved, from the Chief Executive to the volunteers who clean and tend the premises and gardens. Words alone cannot convey the impact or value of this within the community. This book is their story.

Contents

Chapter	Title	Page
	Foreword	6
1	St Francis	8
2	The History of the Hospice of St Francis	10
3	Celebrating The Hospice of St Francis	14
4	A Special Place	95

Foreword

Julian Ashbourn was inspired to embark on this project after experiencing our care first hand both at home and in our inpatient unit. His vision of the care we provide offers an insight into the reasons why The Hospice of St Francis holds such a special place in the hearts of so many patients, families and volunteers.

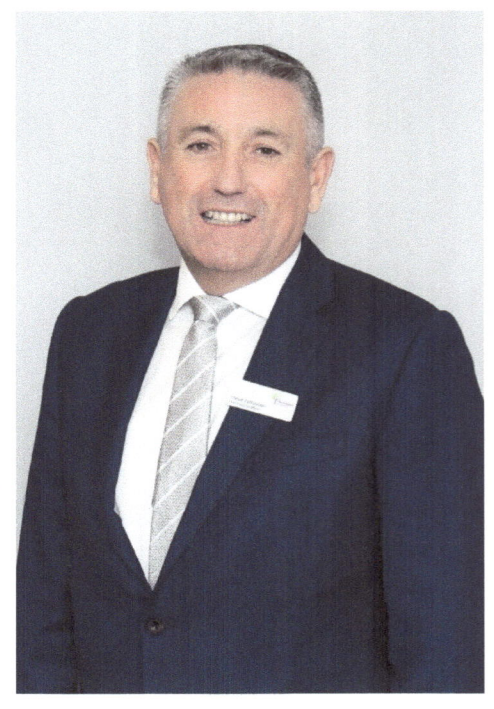

The Hospice of St Francis is so much more than the bricks and mortar of our building. It is the people and volunteers who work here who embody the values, principles and ethos of care that define our organisation. It is the combined experience of everyone who comes here. It is the services we give to our community, be that in our inpatient unit, in our Spring Centre, in people's homes, or in care homes and hospitals. It is the education and training that enables our values to spread even more widely.

These pages give a glimpse of a few of the people and what the place - and all it embodies - means to them, as well as a chance to reflect on the, perhaps, unexpected beauty and peace of the Hospice and its grounds. Seeing the organisation that I am so proud to lead from the varied perspectives of patients, families, staff and volunteers is a privilege and a pleasure, and I am enormously grateful to Julian Ashbourn for all the work he has done to help me see it again through his eyes and those of so many others. I hope that it will give you the same pleasure and some new insights into the care and the values the Hospice holds so dear.

Steve Jamieson, CEO

The Hospice of St Francis

St Francis Hospice is a place
Filled with special light and grace
Nestled in the gardens green
And all the beauty to be seen
Without and yet, within as well
Where all the stories one could tell
Of that heart that beats within
Flowing like a gentle wind
Through all the rooms and corridors
Bringing comfort, peace and more
For those who haven't fared so well
Of all their numbers who can tell
Yet they remain a group apart
Nourished by that beating heart

But this heart is not of mortar made
Though solid as it is displayed
It comes from all the loving staff
Who enter upon our life's path
To illuminate the way ahead
With kindly words so dearly said
The doctors and the nurses too
And all the other people who
Volunteer their precious time
To make St Francis Hospice shine
Like the northern star at night
To guide all those whose paths just might
Gravitate with unseen haste
To this most amazing grace

Julian Ashbourn

1. St Francis

It is fitting perhaps, that the Hospice is named after St Francis. Who better to epitomise the duty of care towards others and the special kindness which permeates the day to day activities of the Hospice? To many, St Francis will be immediately associated with the love of animals and the natural world and this too is reflected within the beautiful gardens of the Hospice where one may gently stroll among the shrubs and trees in the company of birds, just as Francis himself would do.

However, the love of the natural world was but one facet of this most remarkable man. It was his love of humanity that touched so many people in his own time. Indeed, one of his first acts along the road of his conversion was to stop and climb down off his horse in order to kiss the hand of a leper and so bring him comfort. This compassion and care for others when they most need it, regardless of their position *or status in life, represents a further alignment of St Francis with the Hospice.

But St Francis' life was not always so saintly. He was born into a prosperous merchant family in 1182 and, as a young man, enjoyed a pleasure-seeking life of luxury among his wealthy peers. He was astute in matters of commerce and was soon playing an important role in the family business. He also sought to distinguish himself in the honour of battle and fought for his town of Assisi, as well as various campaigns further afield, until he was captured and held for ransom for a year by the opposing forces. Perhaps it was partly this experience that gave Francis time to reflect upon the deeper things in life. In any event, by the time he returned to Assisi, doubts had begun to surface as to his own lifestyle. Eventually, things came to a head when Francis gave generously to a poor beggar, and his father became furious and disowned him. Francis, in turn, renounced all his worldly possessions and favoured position and embraced poverty, devoting the rest of his life to teaching and helping others.

Francis' natural charm and leadership qualities ensured that others followed his example and, very quickly, he had established a following of individuals from all walks of life who similarly embraced the concept of poverty, thus setting themselves free from the cares of material life, confident that God would provide for them. Francis considered that his brotherhood included all of God's creatures, animal and human alike, and initially had no thought of establishing a Holy Order. However, it became clear that his followers were steadily increasing in number and Francis understood that he must bring some structure to the situation, eventually establishing the Order of Poor Ladies which was later called the Poor Clares.

It seems that everywhere he went Francis inspired others with his devotion to the poor, needy and sick and his appreciation of the natural world. Seldom has one man exerted such an influence so long after his own passing. Furthermore, it is an influence which transcends geography, culture, language and even religion as Francis' teachings are universal and strike a chord in every receptive heart.

This ethos of care and kindness towards the sick and those who might otherwise face trying times alone was at the heart of Francis' life and teachings. How fitting then, that his name should grace The Hospice of St Francis and continue to inspire all those who come together to make the Hospice such a truly special place. A place maintained by the loving care and efforts of the individuals involved, just as Francis' own followers brought peace and comfort to others in his name. Indeed, the tradition lives on as though St Francis himself were quietly exerting his influence within this little corner of Berkhamsted. It is fitting that we remember him as we walk quietly among the beautiful gardens and care for those who find themselves in need.

And so, as you journey through the pages of this book and discover what lies at the heart of The Hospice of St Francis, think of the journey that was the life of St Francis himself and how his example is reflected even now, as you will realise with every turning page.

2. The History of The Hospice of St Francis

It all started in June 1979 when, at a special prayer meeting at St. Peter's Church in Berkhamsted, the need for a local hospice was identified, and a commitment made to establish such a facility. Some funding was raised and the Sisters of St Francis offered the use of their convent in Shrublands Road as an initial base. This turned out to be providential, not just in the naming of the facility but, in 1982, the Sisters were recalled to their Mother House and the property in Shrublands Road came on to the market. On 1st September 1982 the property was duly purchased and a programme of refurbishment initiated.

Various funding activities were undertaken and the residents of Berkhamsted proved generous in their support of the new venture. In 1984, the Day Hospice opened on Tuesdays and Thursdays and was able to accommodate eight patients each day. This was followed in 1986 with the opening of the Inpatient Unit which comprised three single rooms, a double room and a triple room. This was an exciting time for all those involved to see the beneficial impact that this was having on the community.

The Hospice continued its good work and, before long, it was evident that more space would be required. The house adjacent to the Hospice was bought and this provided space for enhanced facilities. Care at home for patients was also introduced, widening the impact that the Hospice was to have upon many lives. In 1999, the decision was made to build a new Hospice and the search for a suitable site began. In the meantime, administrative offices were opened in Church Lane and Kings Road.

In 2001, the site at Shootersway was identified and, when in 2003 planning permission was finally granted, the site was purchased with a legacy from Mr Paul Beard. During an early visit to the new site, it was reported that an unusual double rainbow appeared, as if in blessing of what was to come. As 2003 became 2004, plans moved forward swiftly, with a Project Manager appointed and, in June of that year, a detailed design of the new facility finalised. In September, the planning application was submitted. At the same time, an appeal for funding was launched and things quickly moved ahead, with planning permission for the proposed building approved in December, just before Christmas.

Throughout 2005 work continued, firstly below ground and, in November, the above ground works started to be visible. Meanwhile, various funding initiatives were initiated including the Berkhamsted Gazette Dig D££P appeal and, in early 2006, the innovative Big Brick Buy whereby bricks could be purchased for £5 each. It is indicative of the generosity of local residents that all of these appeals were warmly responded to. By November 2006, the Kings Road staff were able to move into the new building and, on 18th December, there was a candlelit procession and blessing prior to preparations for the Day Hospice.

January 2006 was a busy time with the Day Hospice becoming operational and staff moving in from the Shrublands Road site, which was then closed. On 15th January, the Spring Gardens building was certified by the Healthcare Commission and, on 22nd January, the first patient was admitted. All the while, administrative staff were working hard to ensure that funds would be available to sustain the operation of the Hospice.

In 2013, The Spring Centre was opened to offer additional support for patients, families and carers, and has proved to very successful. Indeed, The Hospice of St Francis has been flourishing in all respects, providing a much-needed and appreciated level of care, which would otherwise have not been available within the community. The benefit for patients is incalculable and provides much more than just clinical support. The palliative care and concern for patients *and* families is of the highest order and well above expectations.

None of this would have been possible without the dedication of the staff and volunteers or the generosity of local residents who continue to support The Hospice of St Francis, which stands as a testimony to how something quite wonderful can happen when like-minded people come together to support those in need within their community. But the effort is ongoing. We must sustain this unique facility into the future and ensure that the inspiration behind its conception and subsequent development is never forgotten. The Hospice of St Francis is a cornerstone of Berkhamsted itself and long may it remain so for future generations.

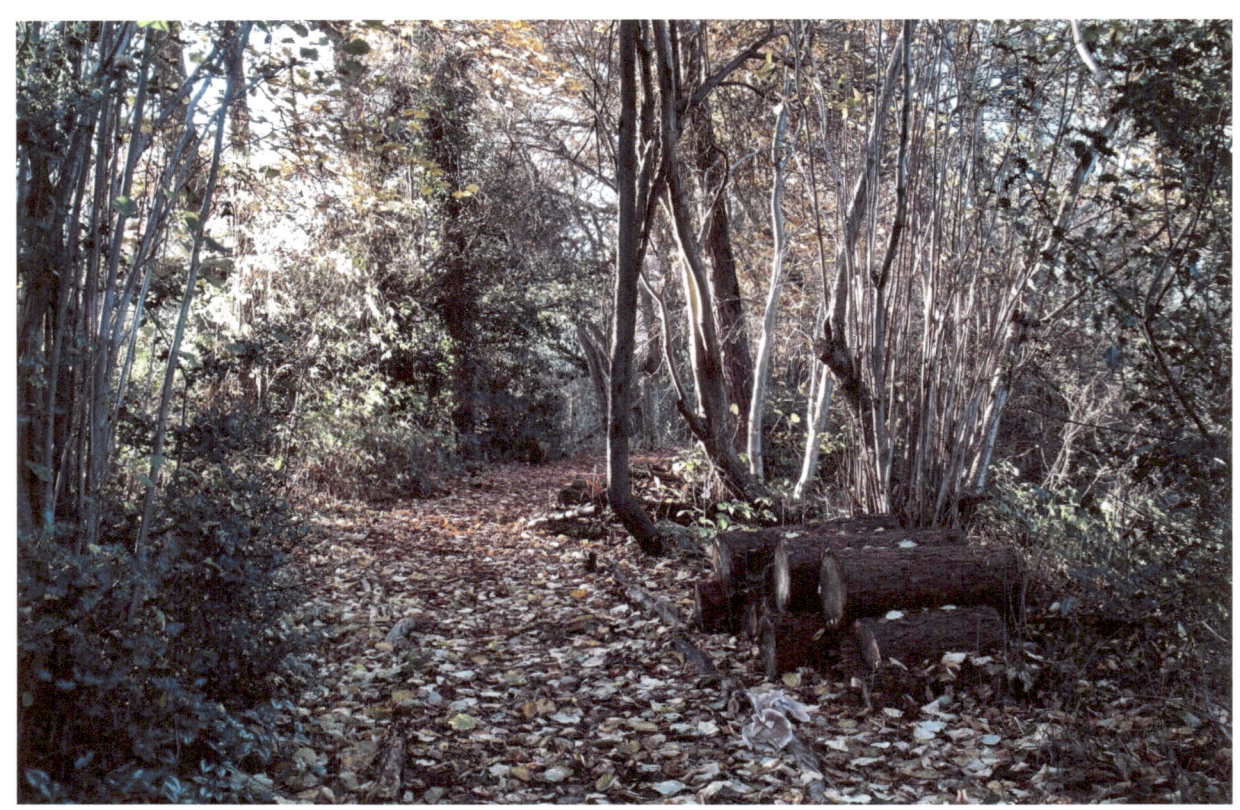

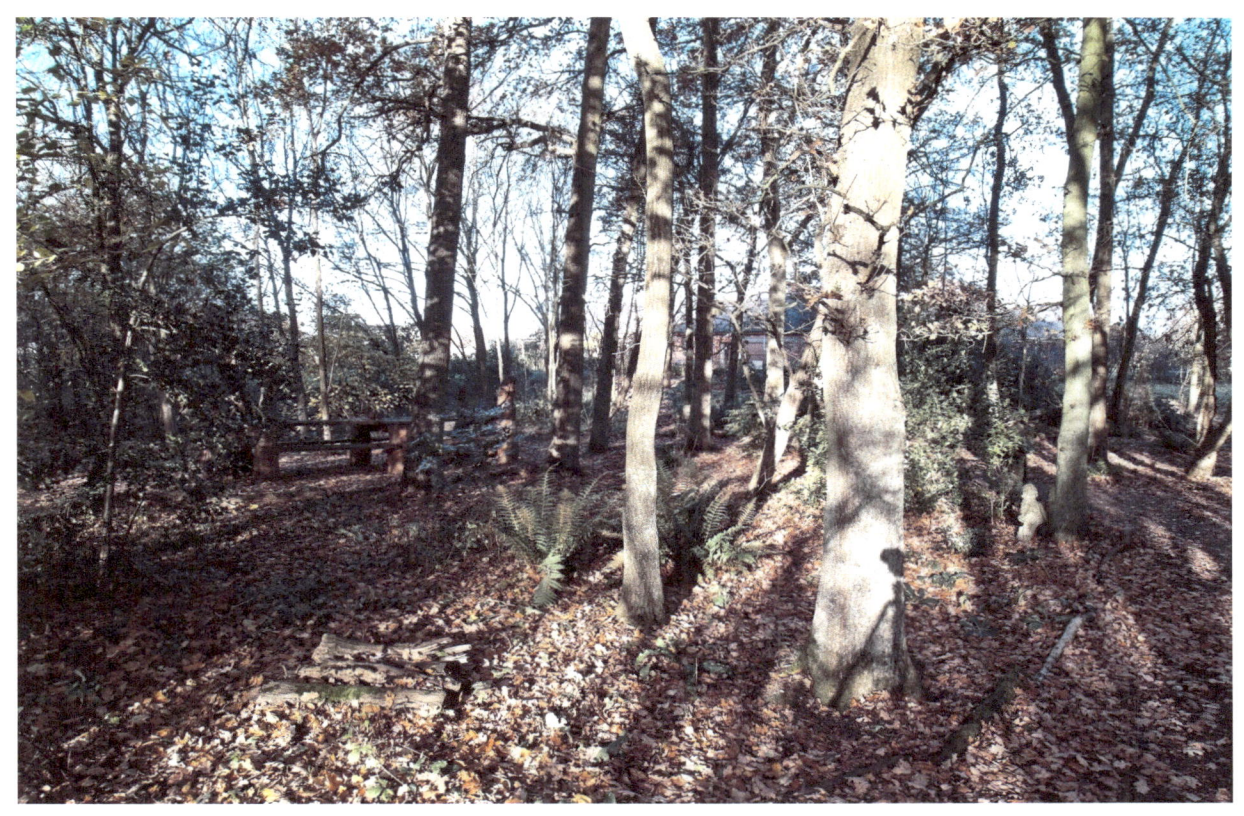

3. Celebrating The Hospice of St Francis

The beautiful woodland path is full of fascinating structures and colours, woven together in nature's beautiful tapestry. The early morning sunlight, throwing its shadows across the path as it winds its way mysteriously through the trees, creates all sorts of interesting patterns as it illuminates the woodland floor. Some nicely cut logs, a few young beech trees and a carpet of lovely coloured leaves, provide a glorious setting. Life finds a way, even on the woodland floor and in the leaf litter as these beautiful fungi demonstrate. What wonderful, delicate construction which seems to come from nowhere. A couple of young silver birch trees add to the colours of autumn, and in the spring and summer, this path will be a blaze of colour. At the end of the woodland trail, you come across the steps leading back up to the main lawns.

"The Hospice is very calm and peaceful and it's somewhere that feels like home, where you're surrounded by lovely people, who have incredible expertise and the most empathy of anyone I've ever met."

Rebecca, work experience student

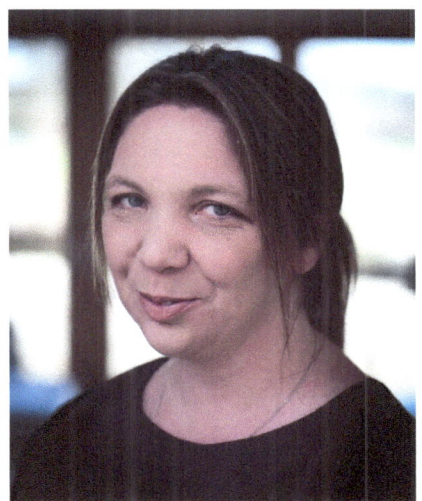

Tania
Clinical Bereavement and Counselling Lead

"I oversee the bereavement and counselling support for the family members and friends of patients we have cared for here at the Hospice. My team, which includes over 50 trained volunteers, takes pride in providing tailored support to each individual we see. I love all of my work. I am passionate about working with people and supporting them to find a way of living with grief and manage the changes it means for their world. I love working with such dedicated and experienced volunteers, matching them with clients and seeing it work out well. I also love working as part of such a skilled multi-disciplinary team. By providing a space for people to talk about their feelings and giving the right support, we can help to reduce a sense of isolation and worry and alleviate the anxiety and physical symptoms that can be associated with grief. Sometimes talking to someone and having them really listen can be incredibly healing."

The Supportive Care Team extends the care offered to patients and their families beyond the physical, medical care that is so important. Drawing on training in psychosocial care and family work, the range of services offered is broad - ranging from emotional support to practical help with housing and finance, from carers assessments to supportive telephone calls after bereavement, from complementary therapies to creative writing, and more. The support is there, ongoing, for those who need it - and so many say they could not have managed without it.

"I have been volunteering with the Bereavement Support Team since 2014. Volunteering has made me more humble of life and the Hospice is a place of joy even during times of deepest sadness. Within the Bereavement Team, we exchange thoughts and ideas about how to improve our service and how we can better support those who come to us, offering hope to all. Each situation or journey changes my perspective. The Hospice of St Francis has agreed to offer me a placement to work as a Counselling Psychologist (working towards a professional Doctorate in Counselling Psychology). I think my study and my volunteering is a togetherness which feeds from each other. Each experience helps my professional development. My course invites existential therapy and thinking into the therapy room: the bracketing of own assumptions, the being with the client, the phenomenological way of experiencing grief every time anew will help me to step into the client's framework. The training and supervision I receive is outstanding and will help my development towards the professional applied psychologist I would like to be."

Ute, volunteer

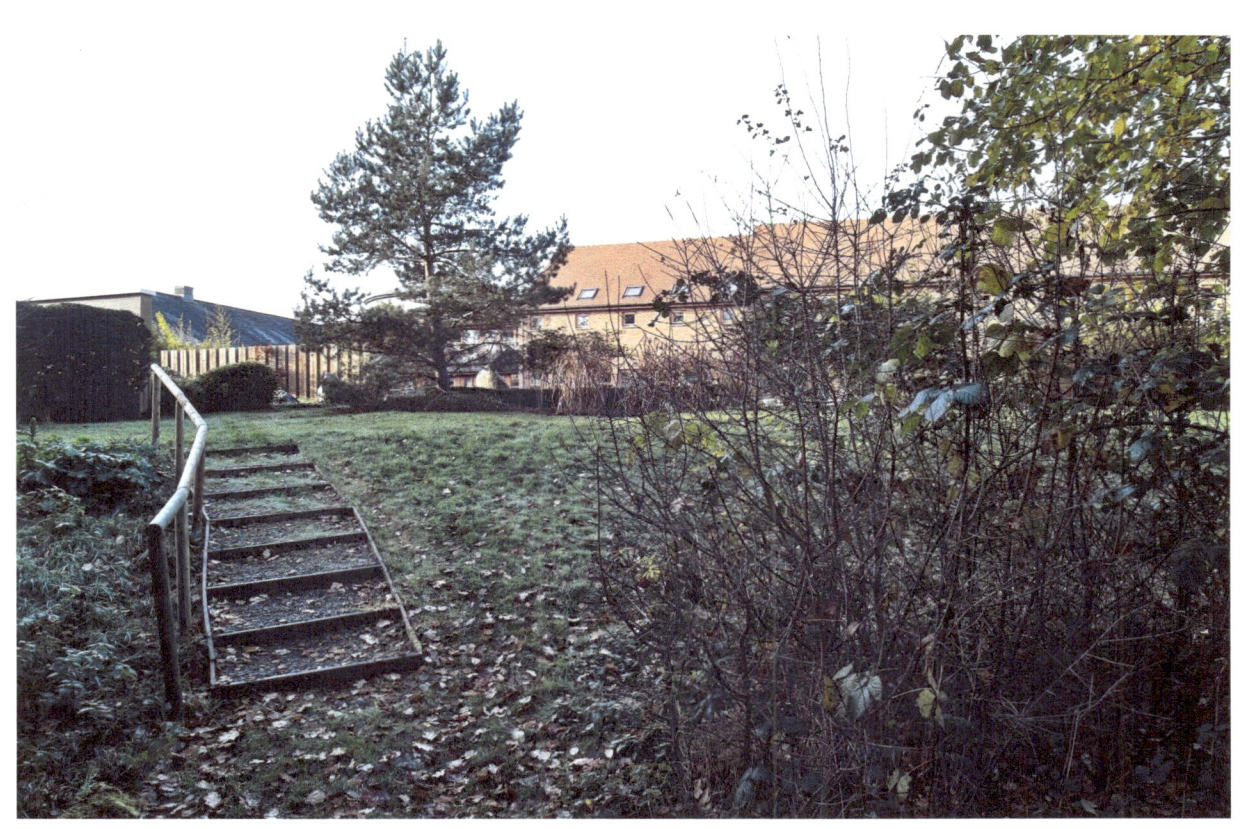

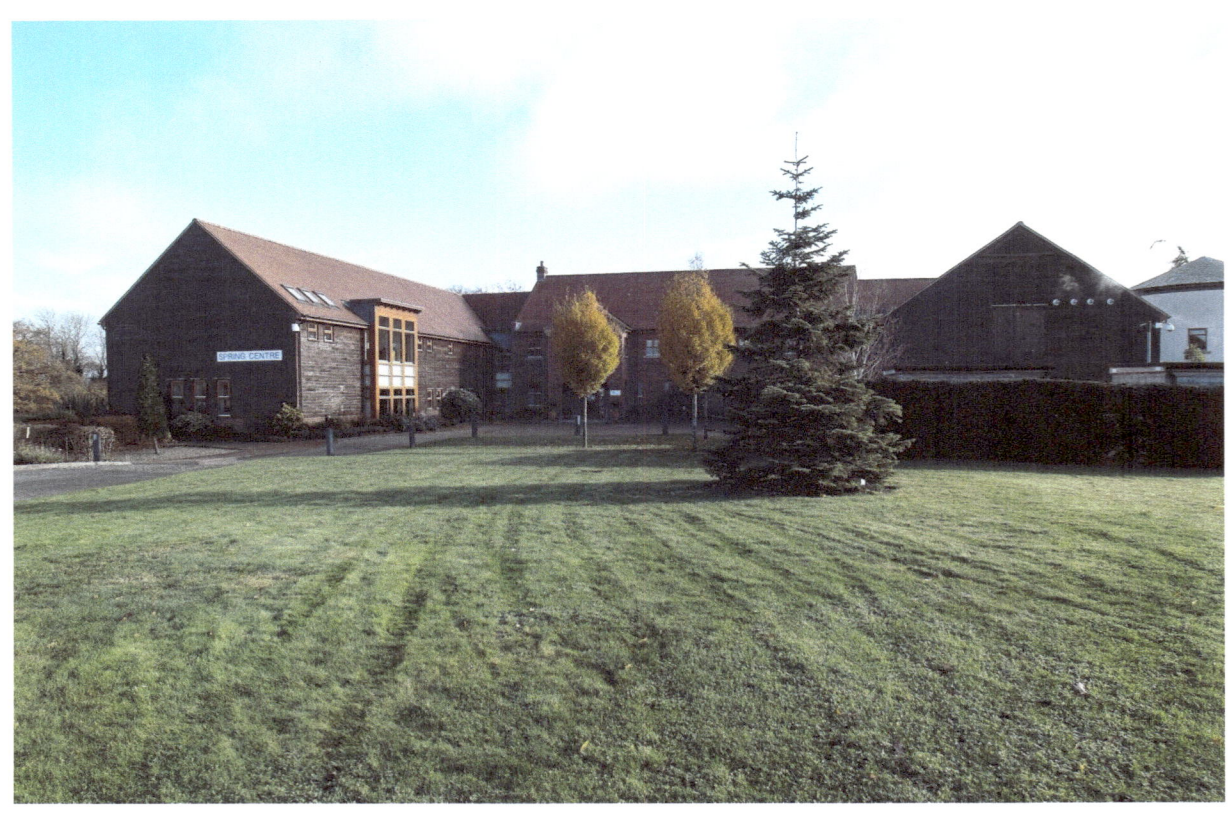

The Hospice buildings come into view as we climb back up from the woodland path halfway along the trail. They may look ordinary but what lies within is extraordinary. The bright morning sun dances around the main building, illuminating and announcing the start of another lovely day. On a fine day, one may sit at one of the many little tables with a view across the gardens to the woodland walk or to one of the ponds. The building houses the Inpatient Unit, the administrative facilities, and The Spring Centre, which has proved an invaluable facility.

"I'm 17 and have applied to study medicine at university. I initially volunteered at The Hospice of St Francis to gain an insight into palliative care, but my experiences there have taught me so much more. Volunteering in the Inpatient Unit, serving meals and chatting with patients, I have learnt the reality that, whilst medicine cannot cure all illnesses, care of the individual can make all the difference in the world. I have seen families spending precious time together in a relaxed and homely environment, sharing meals and memories. The care and compassion shown by all of the staff has been inspirational and has made me realise the importance of seeing the individual and their needs, rather than just the patient and their illness."

Sophie, volunteer

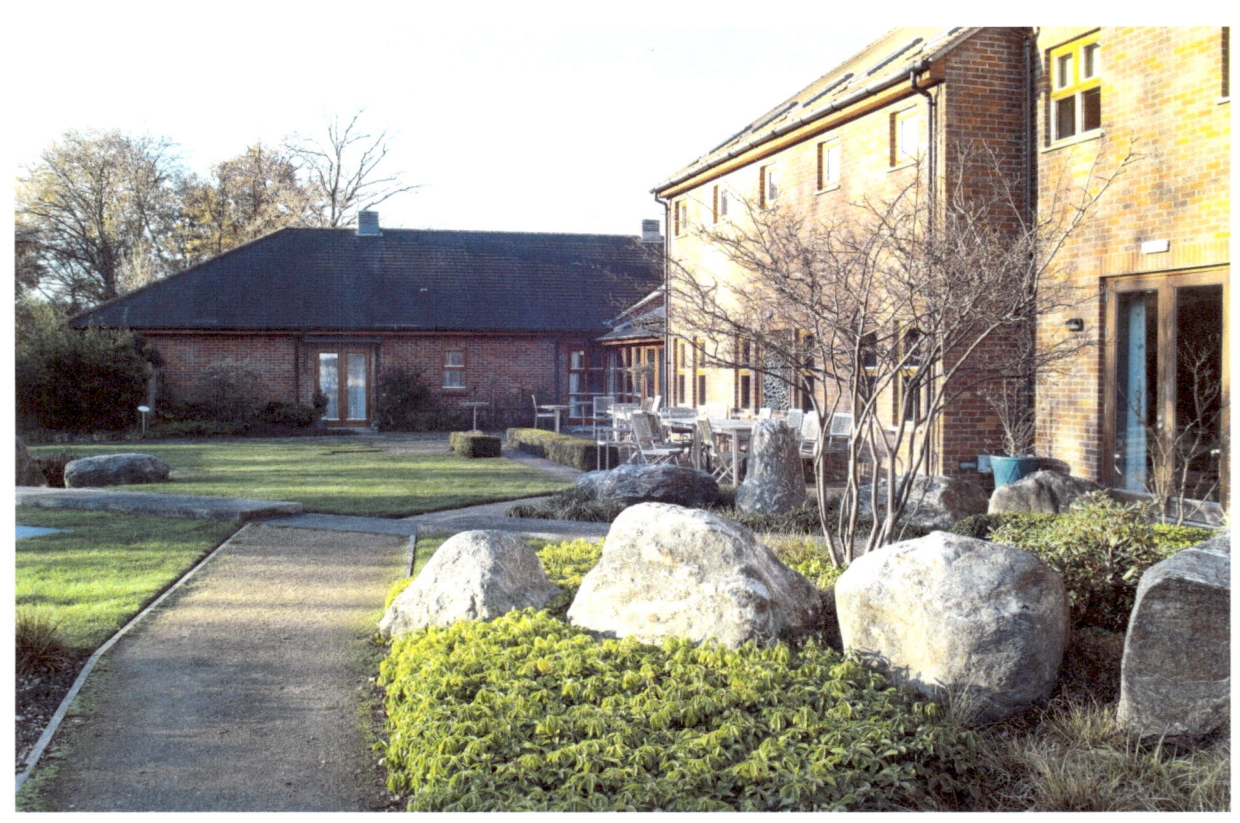

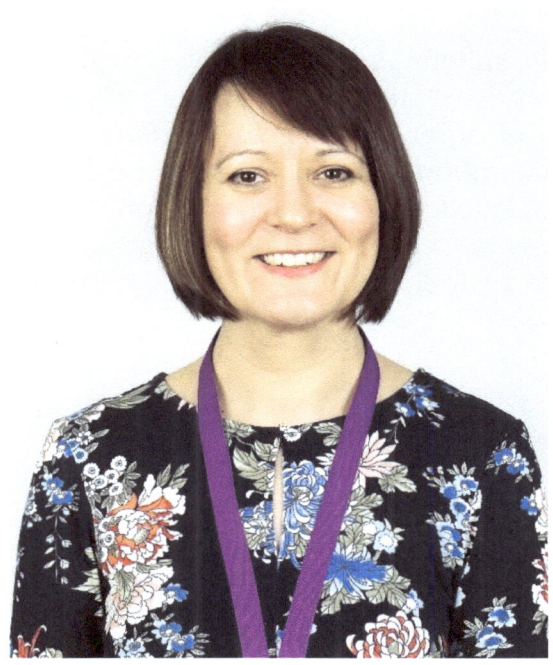

Polly
Senior Social Worker

"I've worked at the Hospice for 12 years and I manage the social work and rehabilitation team which includes physio, occupational and complementary therapists, the carer support team and social workers. My role involves offering psychosocial and emotional support for patients, their families and carers and assessing their social and future care needs. My team and I help to plan care, exploring the support, resources and funding options available - from benefit entitlements and legal services to mediation. The most rewarding part of my job is supporting people to cope with the social and emotional impact that ill health can have on the whole family, helping people to navigate the care system, advocating for people in complex situations and protecting people who are vulnerable and at risk. I really love my job and feel passionate about enabling people to have as much choice and control over their care and situation as possible."

The Hospice of St Francis understands, above all else, that a significant illness affects every aspect of life - not least the practical, day-to-day details that can seem so overwhelming in the face of other challenges. The Social Work team offers support to patients and families, from emotional support to practical help with housing to accessing financial information. For those who are caring for their loved ones, there can be individual carers' assessments to help identify support elsewhere that will fit best with each person's situation. As always, the individual and their family is right at the heart of the Hospice's care.

"Thank you for the amazing care you gave my dad at home and in the Inpatient Unit in the last weeks of his life. The Hospice made the difficult and uncertain process of dying into something which was both positive and life-affirming. As the Operations Director of a charity, I think the thing that impressed me most was the complete absence of any sort of power dynamic in the staff-patient relationship. Staff never used or misused power but completely and consistently gave back to the patient and family. This is so hard to achieve and for it to become the cultural norm, especially within an institution, is truly remarkable. I believe we can all give back by being gentler and more sensitive to all those in need who we meet – ripples that will go out from the acts of loving kindness we received at The Hospice of St Francis."

Ollie, family member

"The place is lovely, but even so is surpassed by the people. The level of care and support is astonishing. The first day here I spent two hours with a doctor talking through my illness and that has been followed up with lengthy daily reviews. The average NHS GP appointment lasts 12 minutes, (although I have a great GP, so mine always go on for far longer.) Yes, I am bored of going through the minutiae repeatedly, but this is critical to ensure that we get a working pain management strategy in place. When I walk out the door at the end of the week, my time here will not have been wasted.

"At every change of shift the nurses and healthcare assistants introduce themselves and let me know who will be looking after me. So far, I have been visited by a social worker, two family support counsellors, a physiotherapist, two chaplains (always my favourite!), the chef, a masseuse, a pharmacist, an occupational therapist, and a partridge in a pear tree. I have probably forgotten someone in my medicated fuzziness, but not only is this team of caring professionals supporting me, more importantly, they are also supporting my family and will continue to do so after I am gone. I haven't even spoken of the army of volunteers, from the garden to the kitchen, without whom I suspect the whole place would grind to a halt. Did I mention that all this is provided free of charge? And that 80% of the funding for the Hospice is provided through charity donations?"

Eamonn, patient

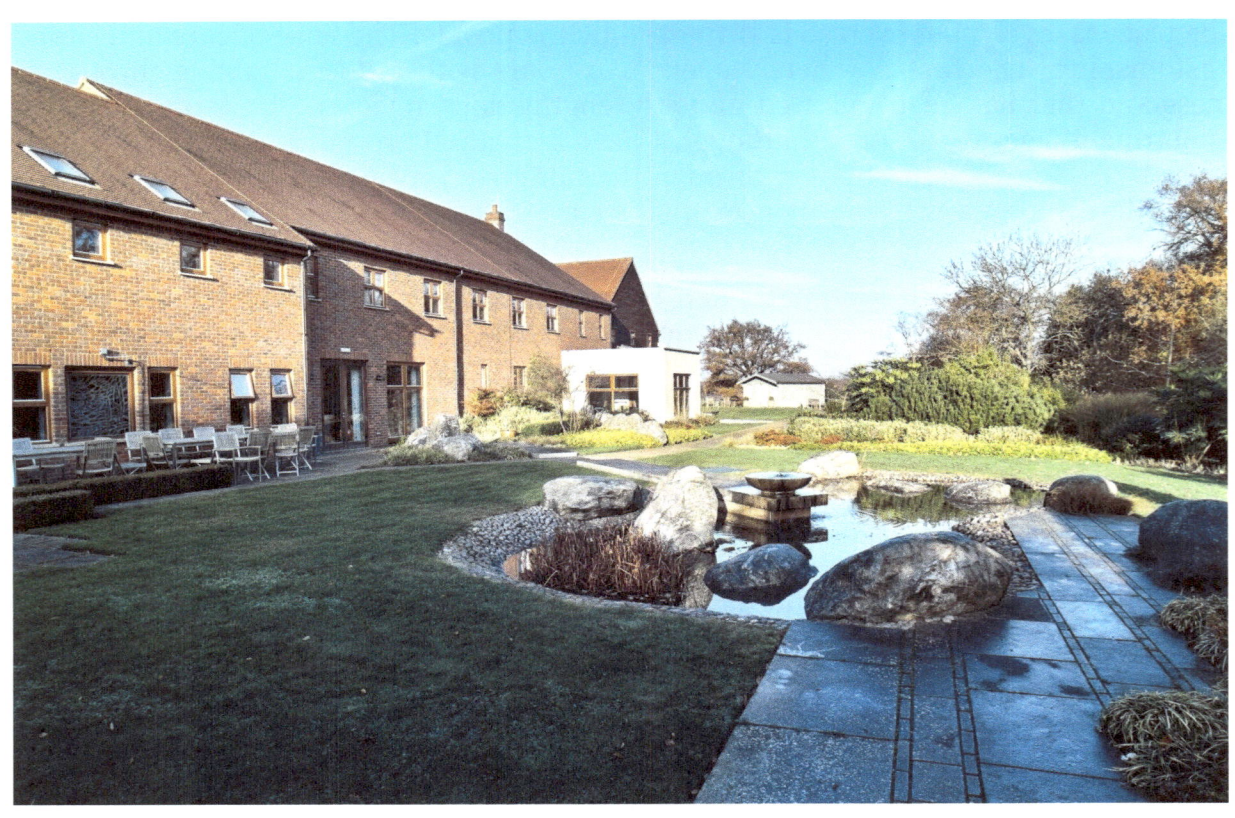

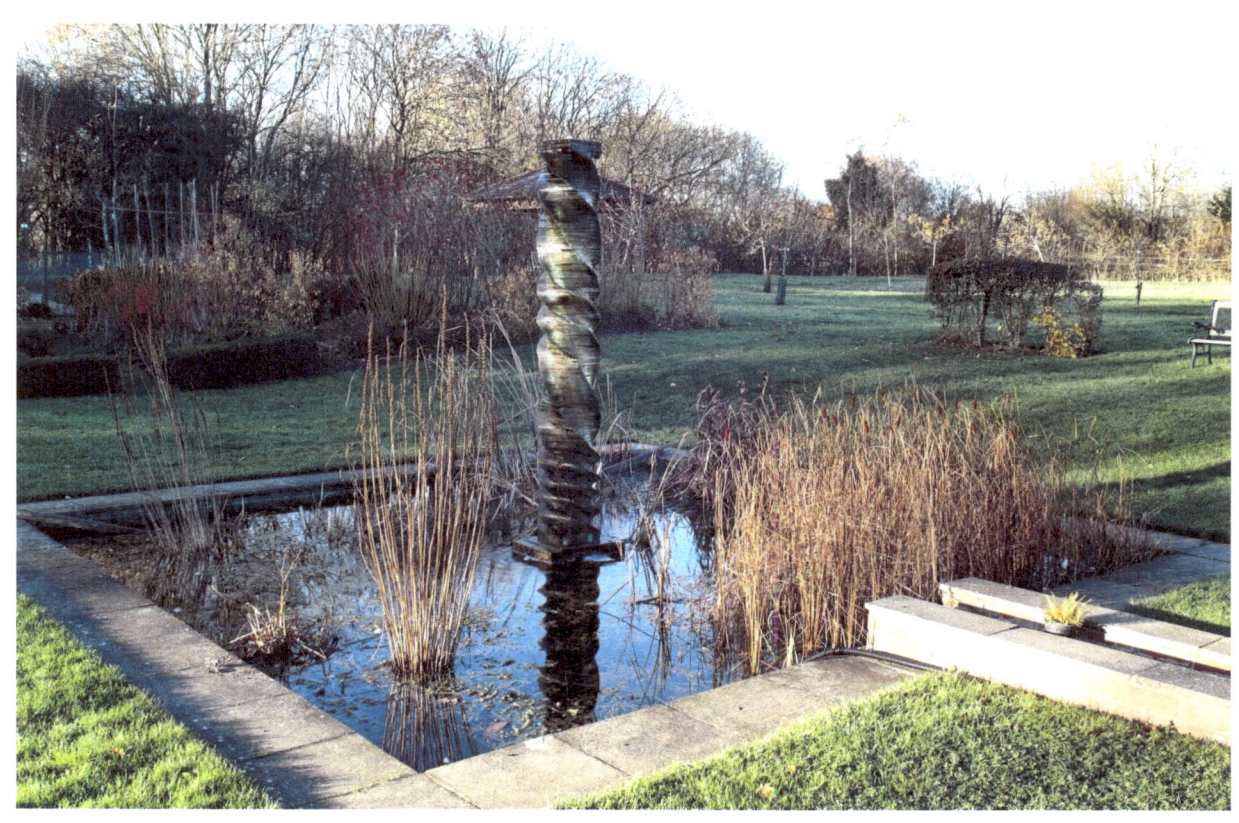

The gardens surround the Hospice, an oasis of peace throughout the changing seasons. Even in the autumn there is a blaze of colour around the ponds set into the lawns for all to see, with little fish darting among the weeds. One of the delightful ponds may easily be seen from the conservatory, the common lounge and other areas within the Inpatient Unit. Another has a most unusual water fountain feature. Interesting shrubs provide a contrast while the trees provide an equally dramatic backdrop. As the hedges are adopting their autumn colours, the trees are shedding their leaves and awaiting their springtime renewal. Even outside there are plenty of little corners where one may sit and rest or chat with visiting friends.

"I think the feeling of being cared for and of belonging for the patients and their families is something that everyone at the Hospice does extremely well. That is borne out by the fact that Florrie continues to enjoy going to Drawbridge and that Tom asked to start going to Teen Drop-in when he found it difficult around the time of Sarah's birthday. They, and I, feel a need to maintain a bond with the Hospice – for whatever reason – and that is probably the best praise you can get."

Chris, family member

"I LOVE it at the Hospice. My team leader is Pam who is delightful, warm and teaching me a great deal. I really enjoy every moment and have met so many terrific people. Thank you for having me!"

Pat, garden volunteer

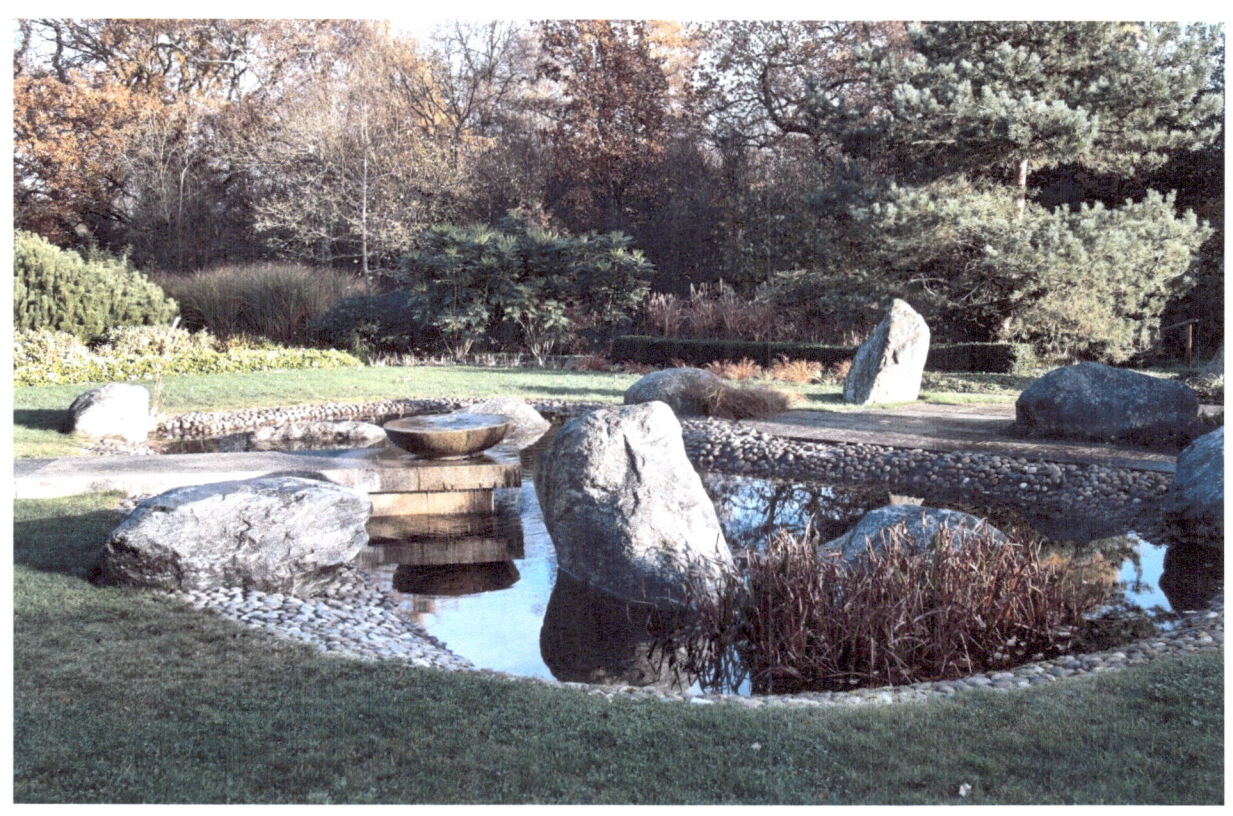

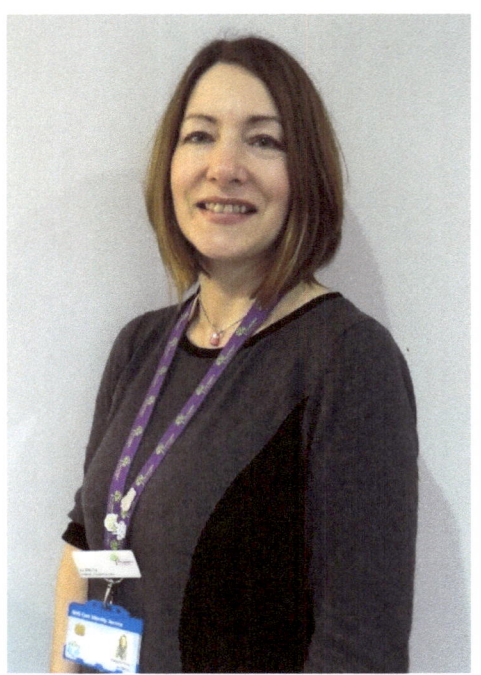

Jo
Children's Support Worker

"As coordinators of the Children's Supportive Care Team, Beth and I work with a team of trained and committed volunteers who provide bereavement support to children, young people and their families and those facing a serious illness in their family. We offer individual and group sessions, as well as family activity and event days. I feel passionate about what I do and privileged that people allow me to enter their lives at very difficult times. When I hear a child or young person saying things like *'So I'm not the only one feeling this then?'* or *'I know now I will have sad times, but I can be happy too,'* then I know the support which our team has given has been valuable. I feel hugely touched to know this and that I have made a difference to a child, young person or adult through a time when they felt lost. I also really enjoy the fun times in my role, such as hearing and being part of the fun and laughter during our Pony and Family Activity Days.

"For a child, understanding a significant illness in one of the 'grown-ups' they love, or the experience of bereavement, can be confusing and overwhelming. The Children's Supportive Care service at the Hospice walks alongside young people in their journeys, encouraging them to express their thoughts and feelings - however hard, however frightening, however unexpected. There may be so much a child needs to ask, but is perhaps afraid to, and the Hospice is a safe, supportive place which encourages reflection and sharing -- through play, through art, through stories, through activities. The regular 'Pony Days' too, offer one more way to share and talk."

"We'd had excellent care in hospital but Paul said the nurses at the Hospice and the care they gave him was beyond anything he'd ever experienced. The care, the love and the support was amazing. Those precious moments like us all having ice cream in his room together and Cordelia appearing on a pony on the patio outside his window. "Hi Daddy!" she called from her saddle. The girls took time off school and we'd sit happily with him for hours on the patio, playing silly games, having a sandwich or doing a crossword. Friends and family were free to come and visit and a couple of his old friends even came to read to him and we watched the England Women's Football Team on TV and enjoyed a beer. I hadn't realized I could stay over but for the last six or seven nights I did stay with him and we'd go to sleep holding hands as though we were in a double bed together. As the end approached, thanks to the Hospice's Children's Services team, managing a situation I'd never have been able to navigate on my own, the girls were so well prepared to the point that they knew when Paul was ready to go."

Eleanor, family member

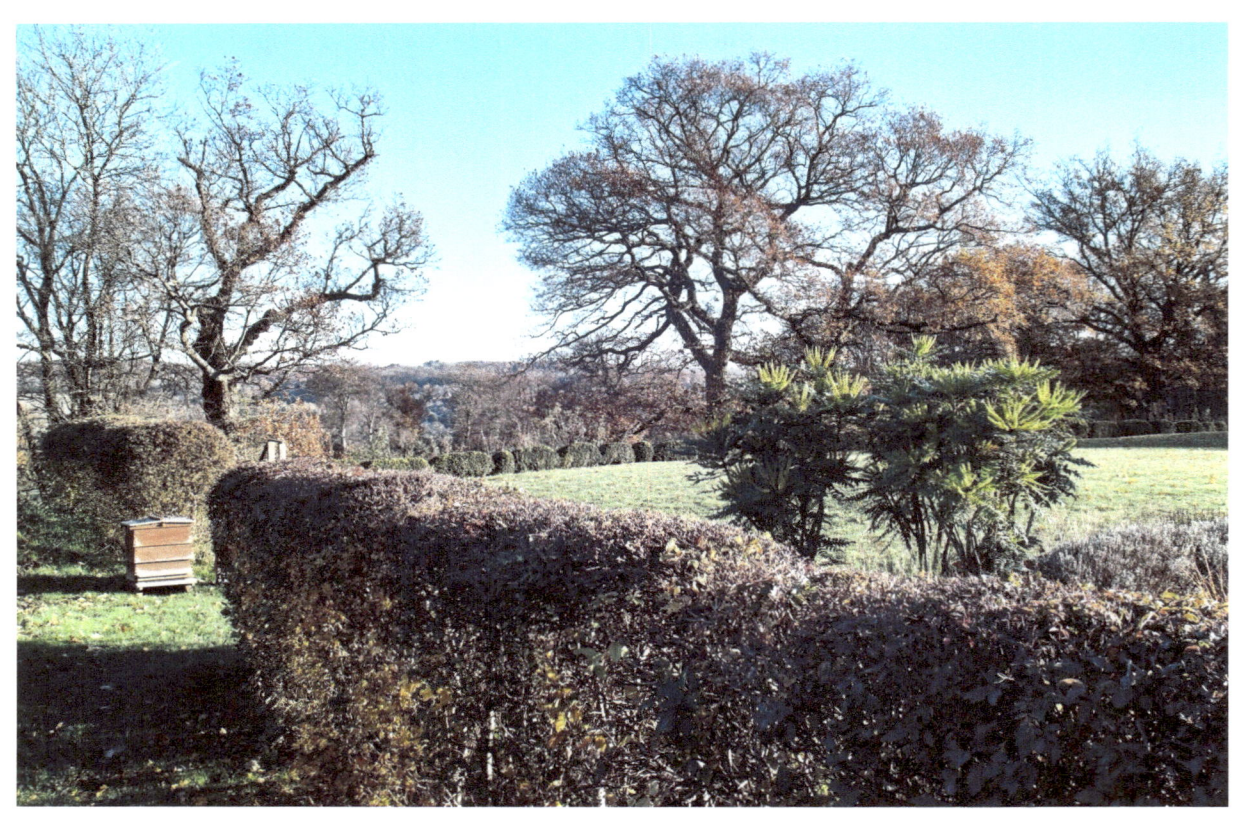

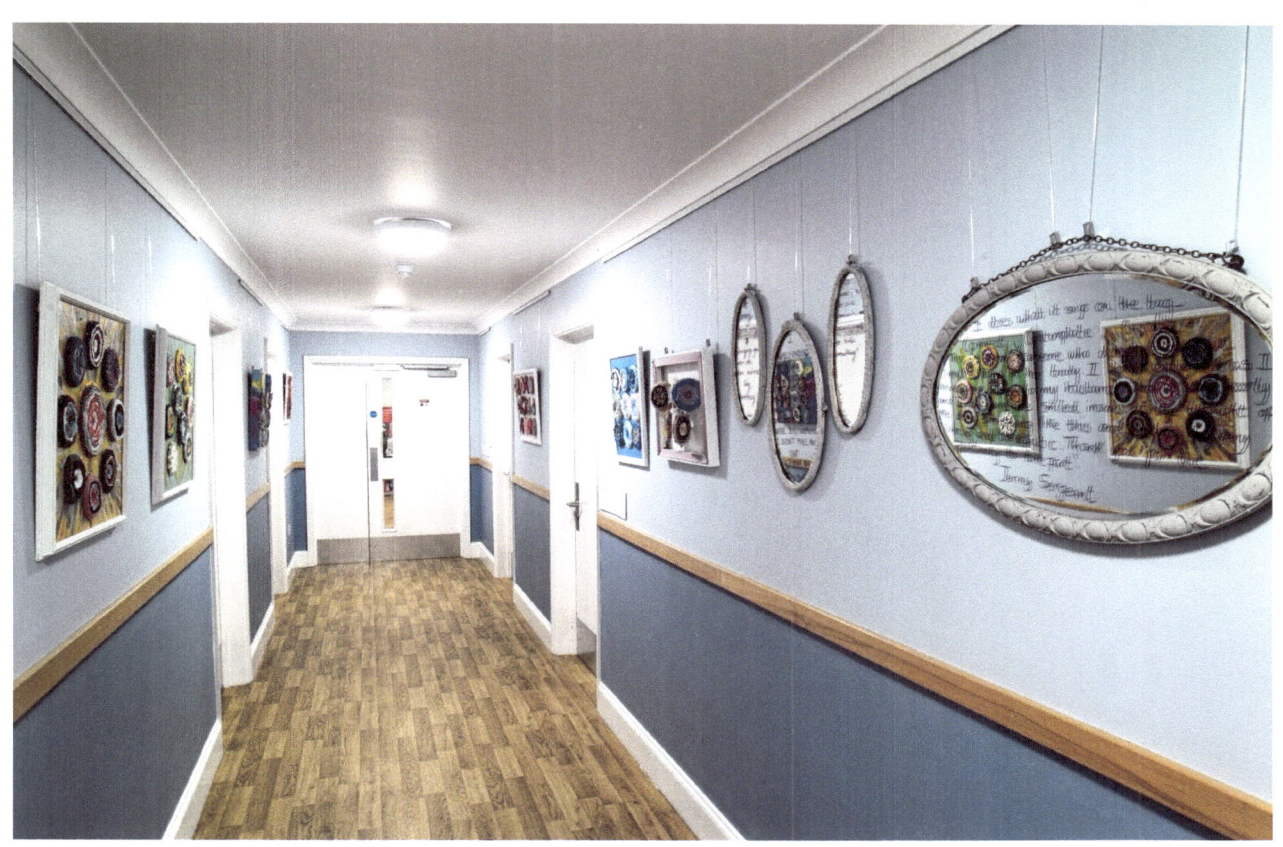

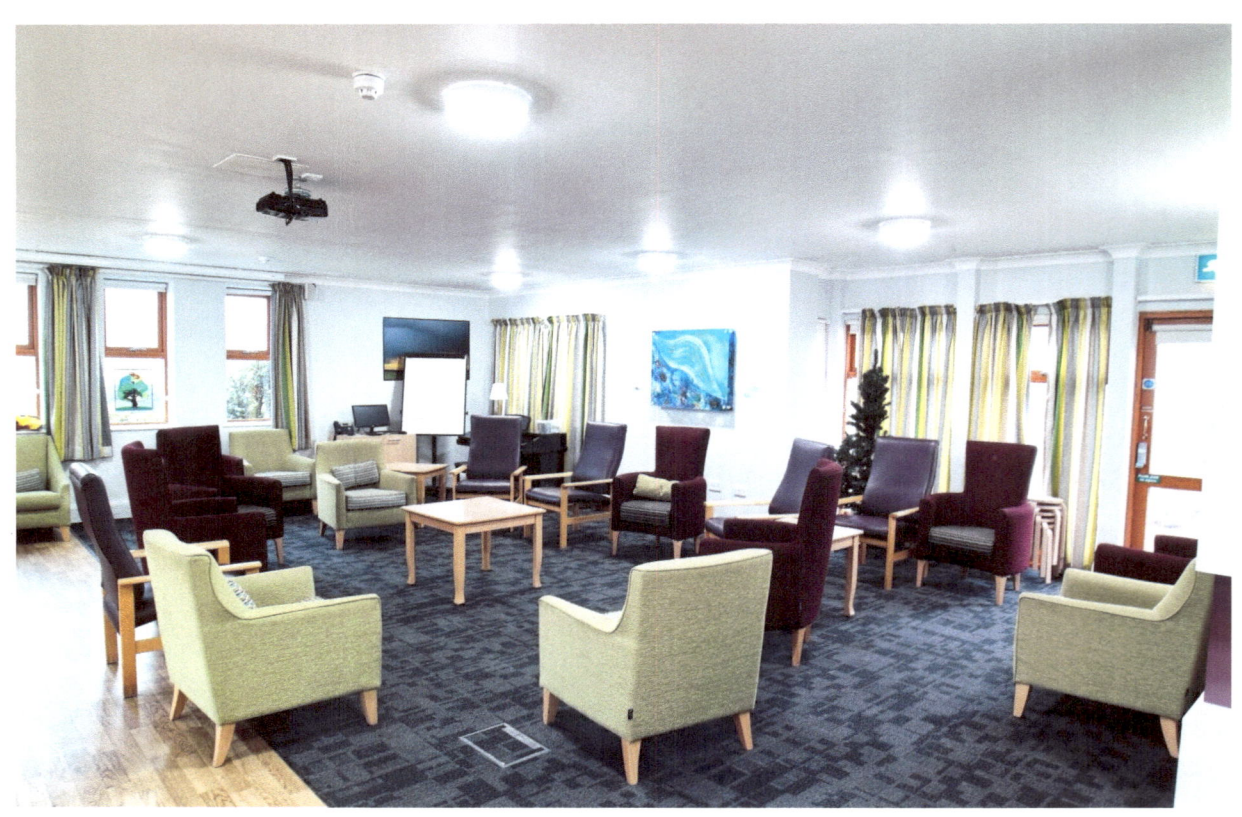

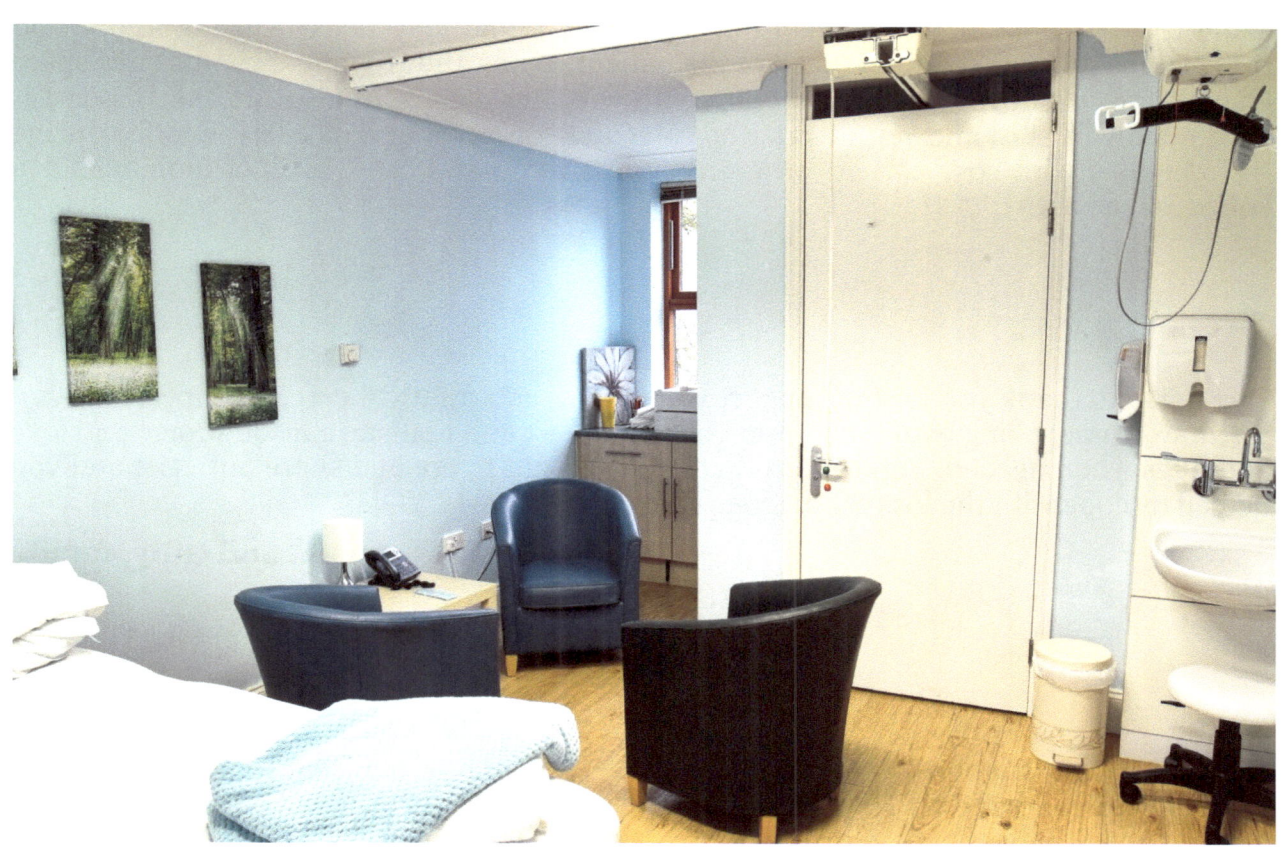

Inside the main building, even the corridors are colourful and cheerful. There are comfortable rooms, filled with natural light, where one may relax in peace and spend time with visitors as required. Each of the patient rooms and treatment rooms have space enough for your loved ones to be there with you. The Bistro area within the Hospice is used mainly by staff and volunteers who can come for lunch or a nice tea or coffee during their breaks, with cosy corners where they can come and catch a quiet moment for a coffee and a chat.

"We'd like to thank you for the support you gave us as a family – care, guidance, always a warm welcome, along with much-appreciated honest and realistic consultations, and love and hugs when needed. You told us that it was alright to cry and share our grief and you helped us cope with the loss of someone dear to us. THANK YOU!"

Alison and Gilly, family

"The all-round support we have received as a family from the Hospice has been invaluable. I can honestly say that our experience has totally changed our perceptions of what a hospice does. It's a really positive place which gave us really valuable time together as a family – time that I will never forget."

Jemma, family member

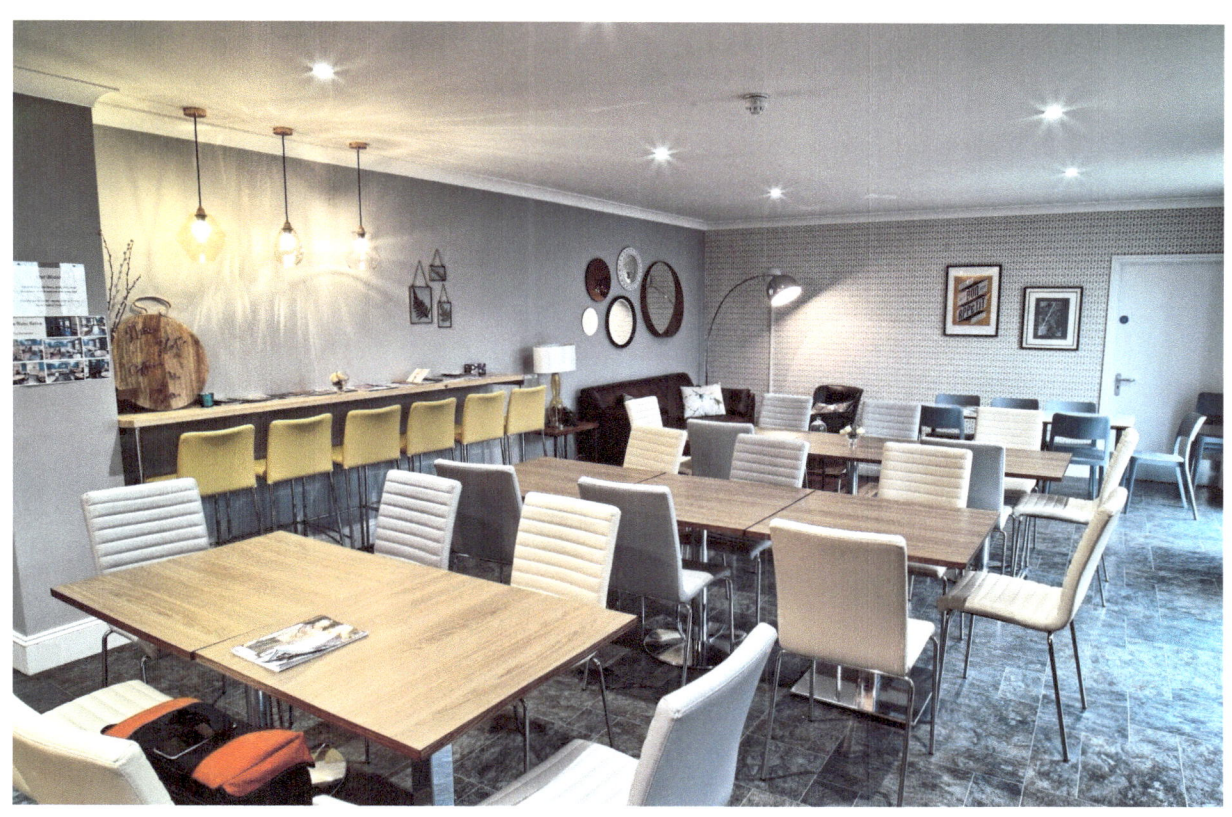

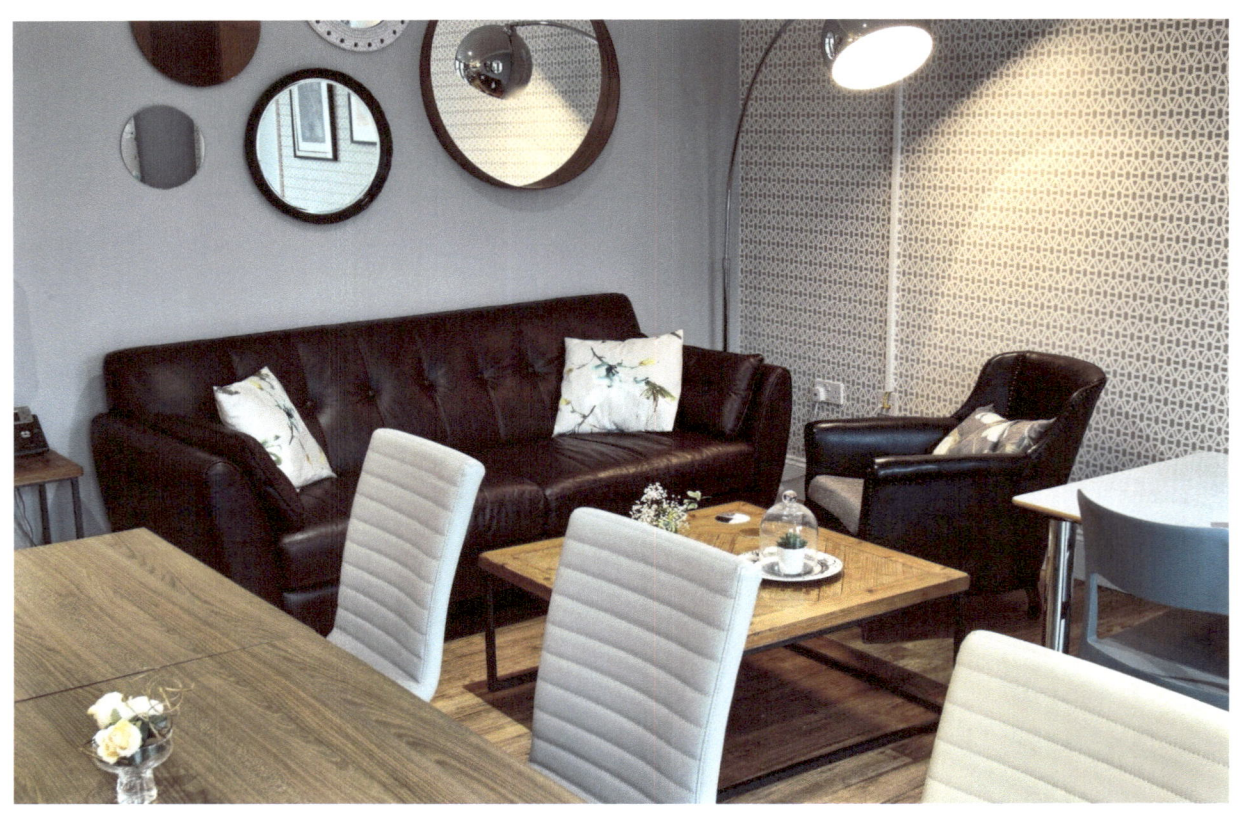

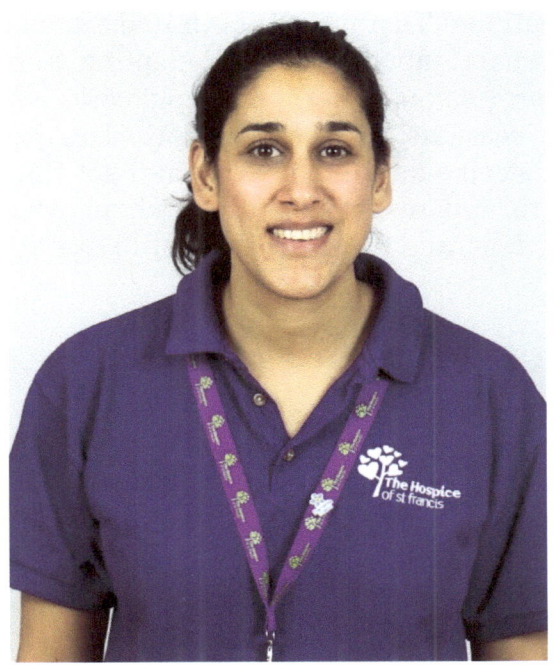

Manisha
Physiotherapist

"As a physiotherapist, I have always been taught to try and fix people's problems; however, working at The Hospice of St Francis, I have learnt that the most powerful tool I have is to educate and empower our patients with new knowledge to enable them to solve their own problems and find strategies that work for them. Our service allows patients to have as much or as little contact as they feel they require. Working with such amazing patients who may be having treatment for cancer, recovering from cancer or dealing with long term conditions has taught me how resilient you can be. I am always so inspired and privileged to be able to help these people on their journey."

Physiotherapy and Occupational Therapy can both make such a difference to fitness and wellbeing, helping with rehabilitation and with adapting to new limits or experiences. Here at the Hospice, the professionals in the therapy teams can work with individuals or groups, offering regular sessions or occasional workshops, problems with fatigue, breathlessness, disturbed sleep - letting you relax and get the rest you need - as well as helping you build strength and resilience. It's all about what each person needs and wants, the goals they hold dear, and the life they want to live.

"Weekly physiotherapy sessions gave me confidence and each week, Sandie would set me small goals to go home, practise and achieve – whether it be making a bed, preparing a meal or washing up. Being able to cook and prepare meals for my family is one of the biggest gifts I have. When I cooked a lentil curry and Safiya, my 13-year-old, said she'd been looking forward to it all day, it was such a proud moment. Instead of feeling like a sick person, I felt like a wife and mum again. I've had so many setbacks along the way but the Hospice has helped me through all of it – I don't know how I would have coped without it. People just need to take more time to understand what the Hospice does and see the positive that comes out of this place. For me it's been the most amazing experience and a total eye-opener."

Wahida, patient

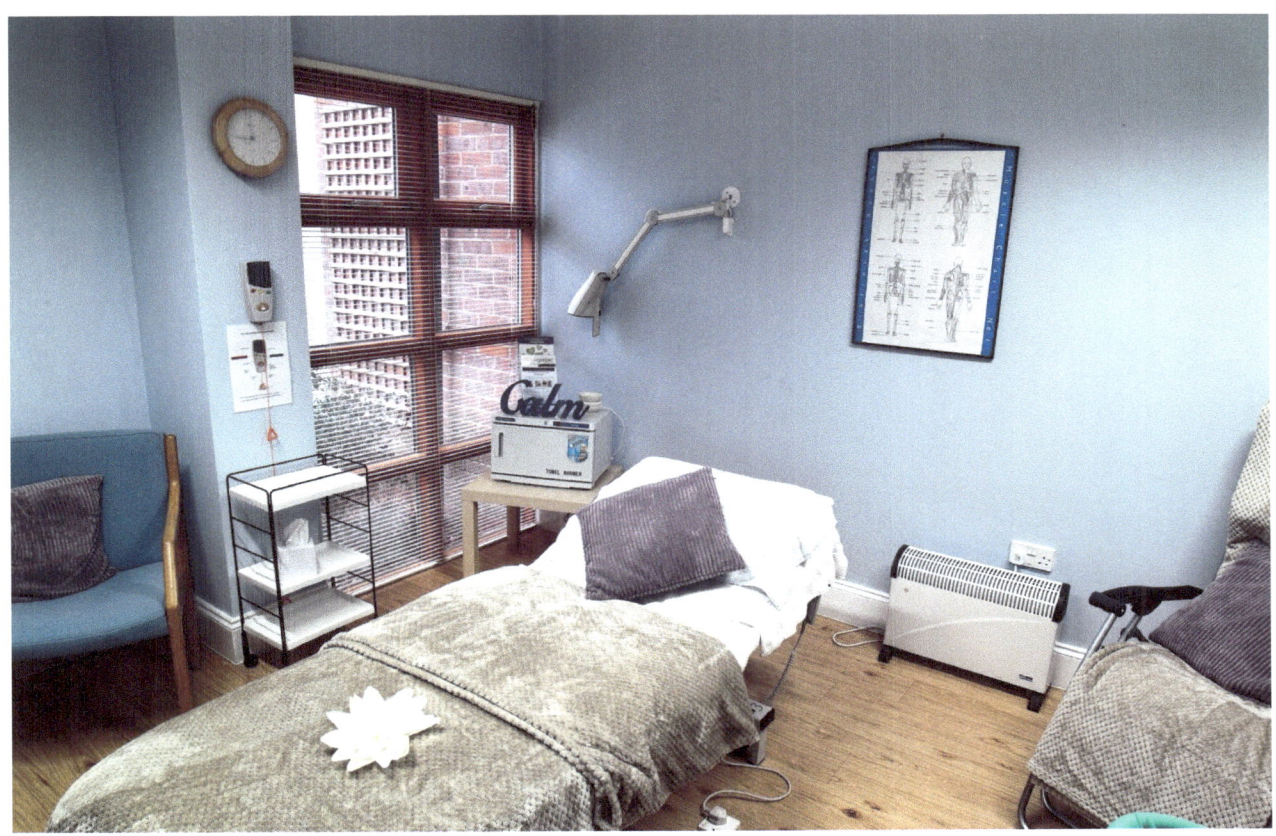

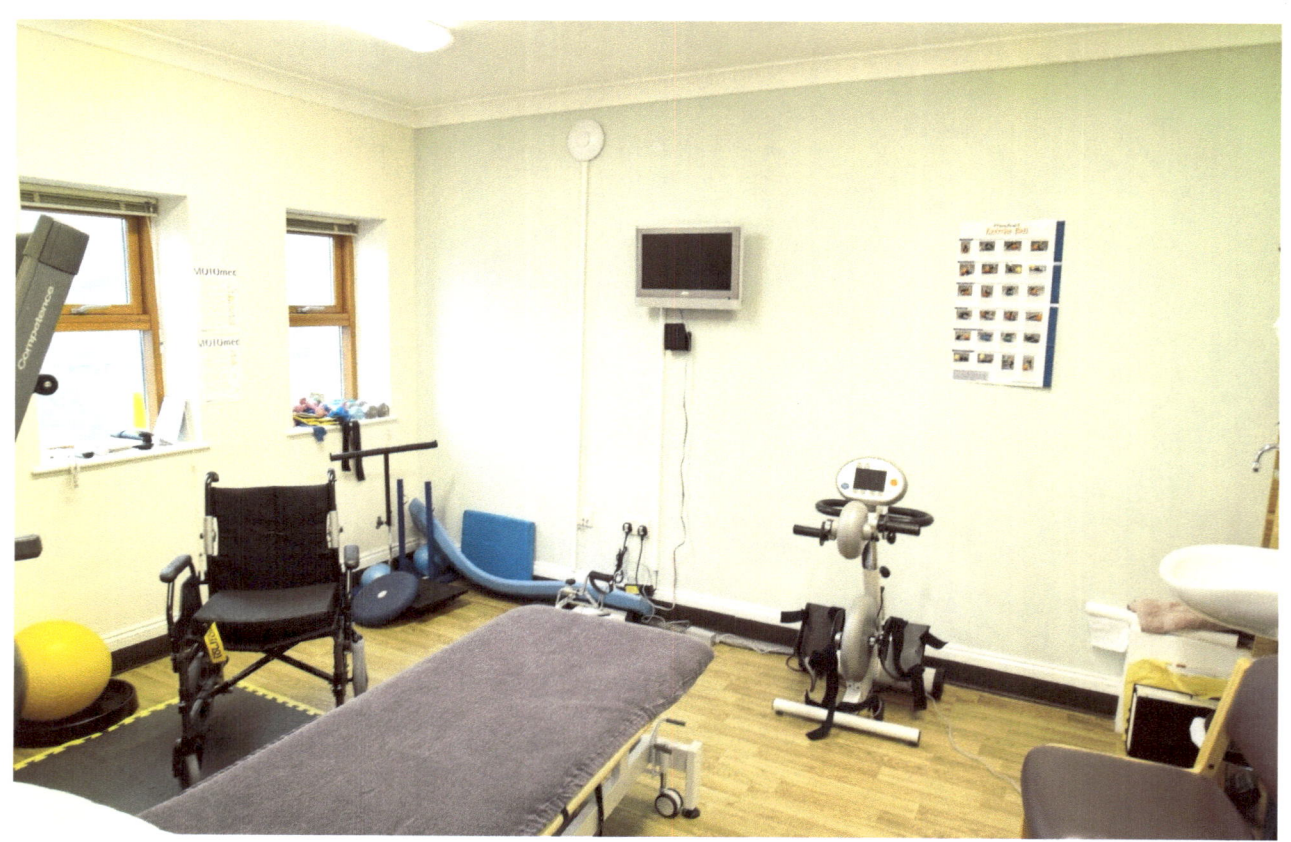

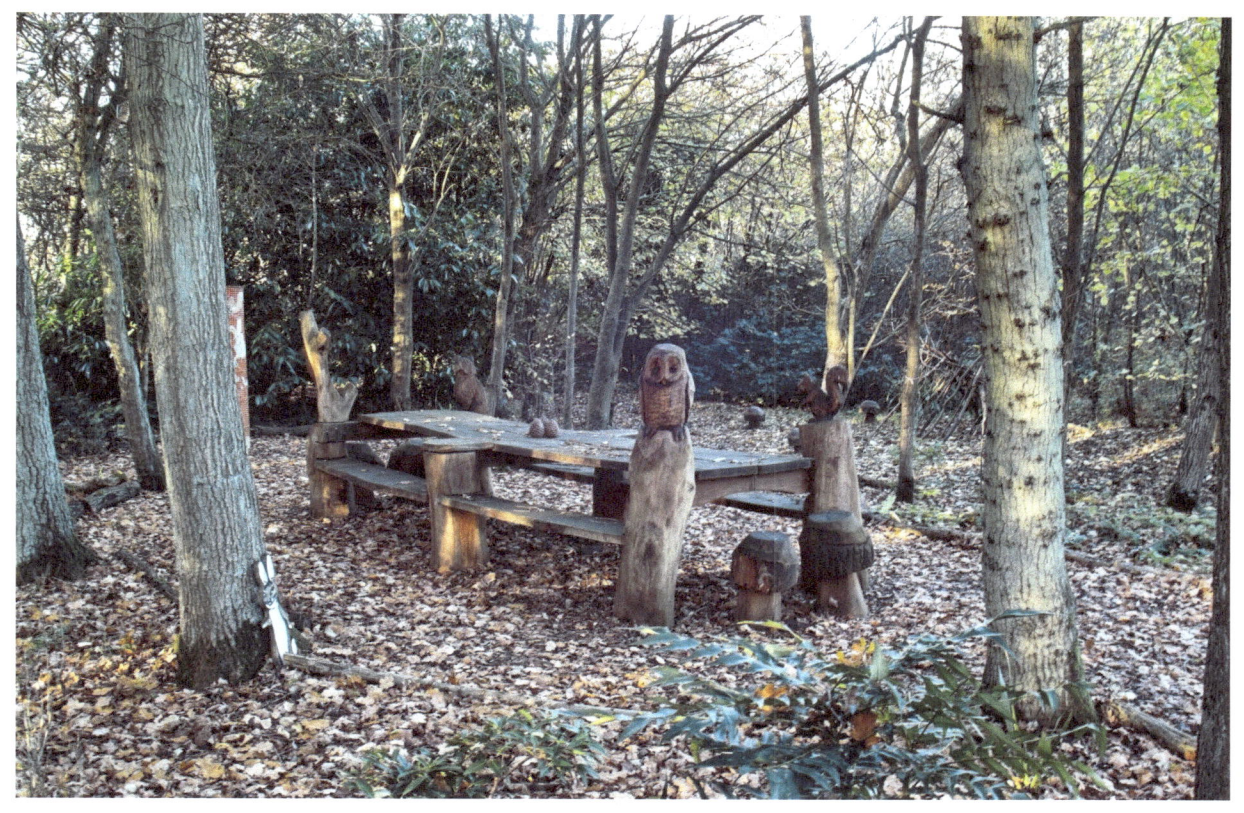

Bertie the bear greets everyone as they descend from the upper gardens to join the woodland path that winds its way through the trees, and keeps watch over the bird tables. Everywhere in the gardens one comes across interesting little corners where, occasionally, one is greeted by a woodland friend. There are places along the trail where small groups may sit and enjoy the company of the woodland. Our friend, the ever watchful owl, pops up in various places along the woodland path and in the clearings - as do so many others, playing joyfully in the morning sunshine amid the colours of autumn.

"I volunteer to say thank you. Joyce, my wife, was diagnosed with cancer in 2002 and Fay, the Hospice nurse, visited us every week for seven-and-a-half years. Joyce had a round - collecting homeboxes for the Hospice - and I took it on after she died. I'm now a coordinator for some of the other collectors. Basically, I do what I can to say thank you."

Tony, fundraising volunteer

"It's not the professional way of giving a service for which people are trained. It's the manner of giving. You stand here for two minutes and someone says 'Can I help you?' and they mean it. There's so much love here - I'm just amazed. I always thought our hospitals were wonderful but this is quite different."

Fred, family member

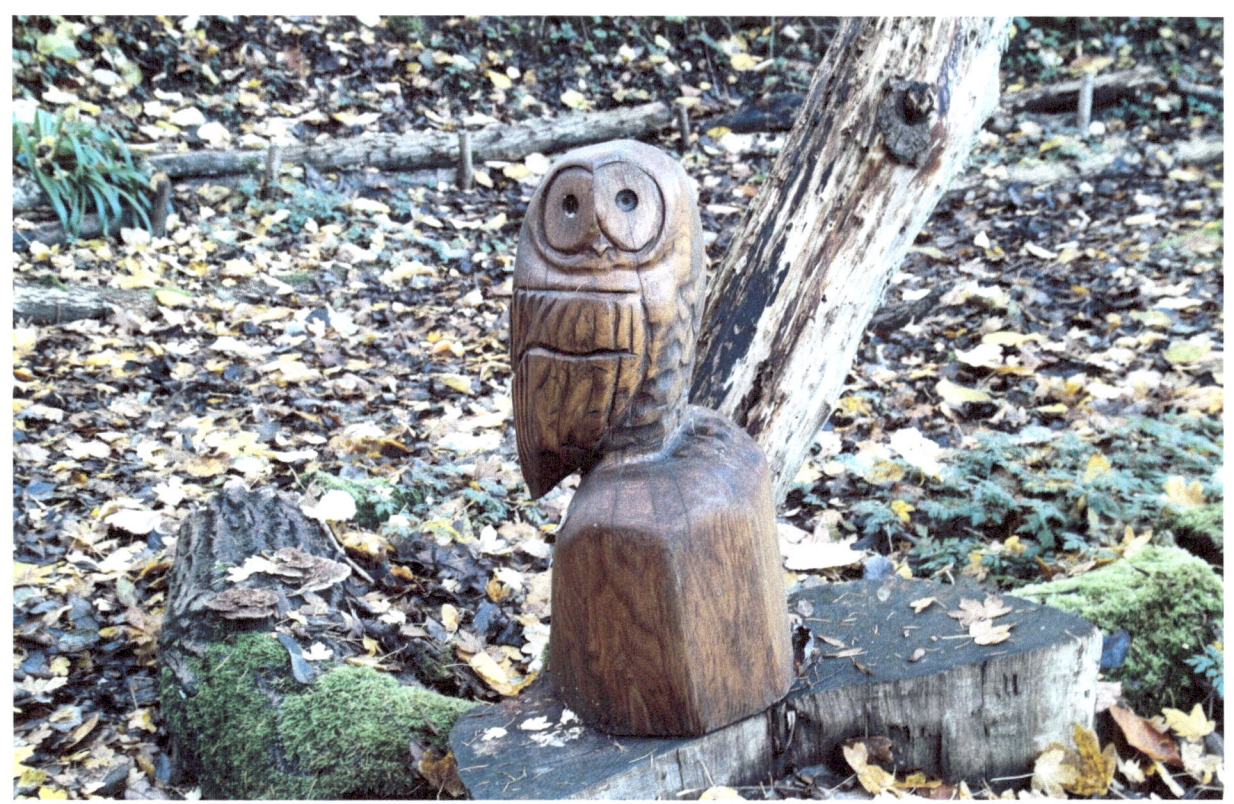

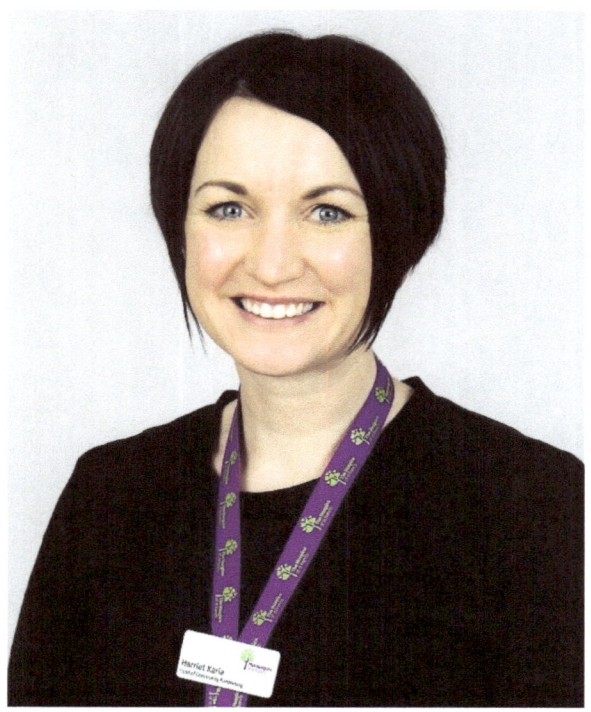

Harriet
Head of Community Fundraising

"Once you start working here, The Hospice of St Francis gets into your blood! I feel so passionate about the care we provide to patients and their families when they need us most, and that drives me and my team to raise the income to fund our work. Working here, at the main Hospice, means that I see where the money we work hard to raise goes and what a difference it makes. I also love the variety of my role: one day I'm knee-deep in budgets and the next I'm meeting someone who has gone that extra mile for us because we have supported their family or friend. I love meeting different people and supporting them on their fundraising journey as I know, both personally and professionally, the impact our care has not only on patients but on their entire family, friends and colleagues and importantly that life is precious and we should live it to the full."

The first idea for a hospice in Berkhamsted prompted a series of fundraising events -- 'snowball' coffee mornings - and the new building, now 10 years old, was only possible through the generosity of hundreds of donors. The Fundraising team is based upstairs, but their work extends throughout the building and the community. From organising huge public events to receiving donations of all sizes from individuals, their work is vital to maintaining and developing the care provided by the medical, nursing and supportive teams. Without the generous donations and fundraising efforts of the wider community, the Hospice simply would not be here.

"I'd heard about the Hospice and its fundraising events but I'd never really understood what it was for. I couldn't believe somewhere like it existed and that I was lucky enough to be in it. I can never thank the Hospice enough for helping me heal at such a critical time in my recovery and giving me back my life. Without it, I don't know what I'd have done. The Hospice has never failed to continue its care for me."

Charlie, patient

"It's hard to explain how grateful we are that Dad spent his final days at the Hospice, which transformed the last 10 days of his life and our last days with him. It really was a little bit of heaven before his passing. A year ago, if you'd asked me to donate to a hospice, I probably would have said there are more worthy causes for people who are going to live. However, now that I've seen the effect this Hospice had on Dad and on our wider family, I am converted. This special place helped us make the most of Dad's final days and we are eternally grateful to all the team at The Hospice of St Francis."

Brian, family member

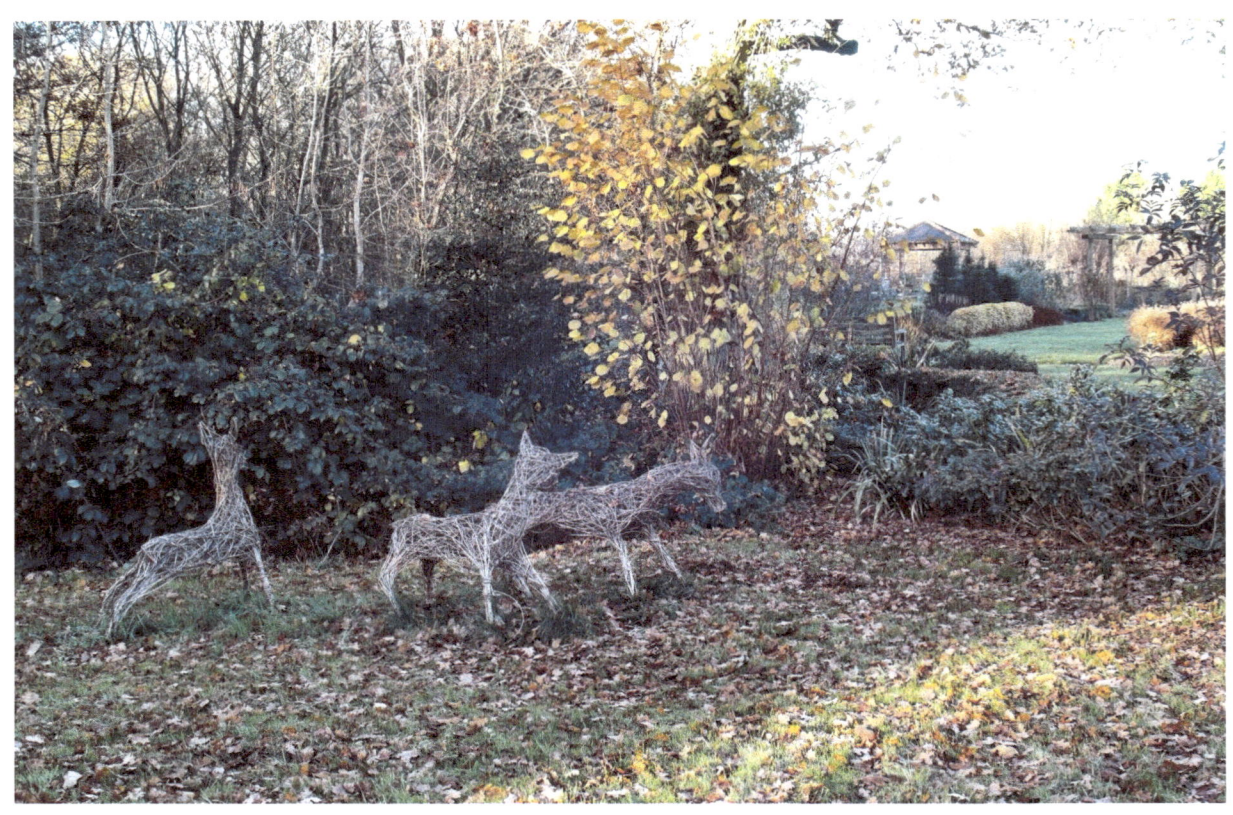

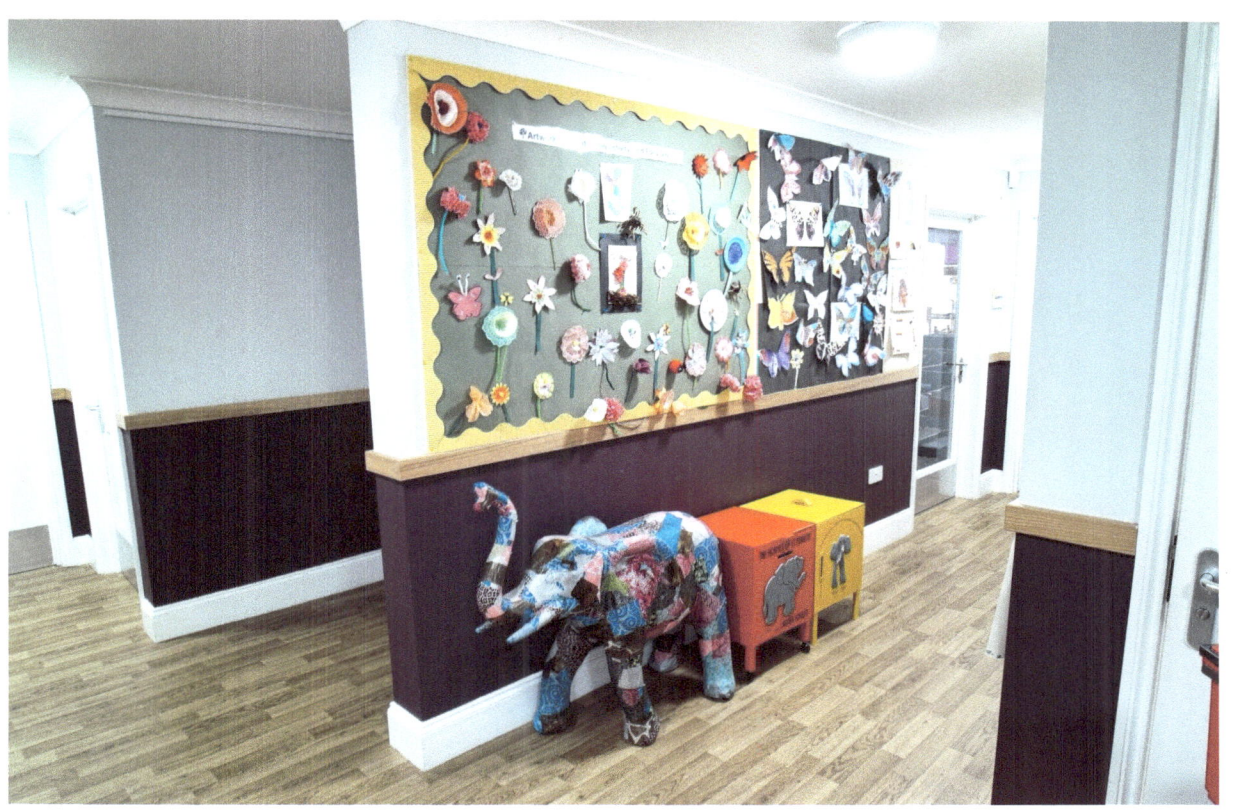

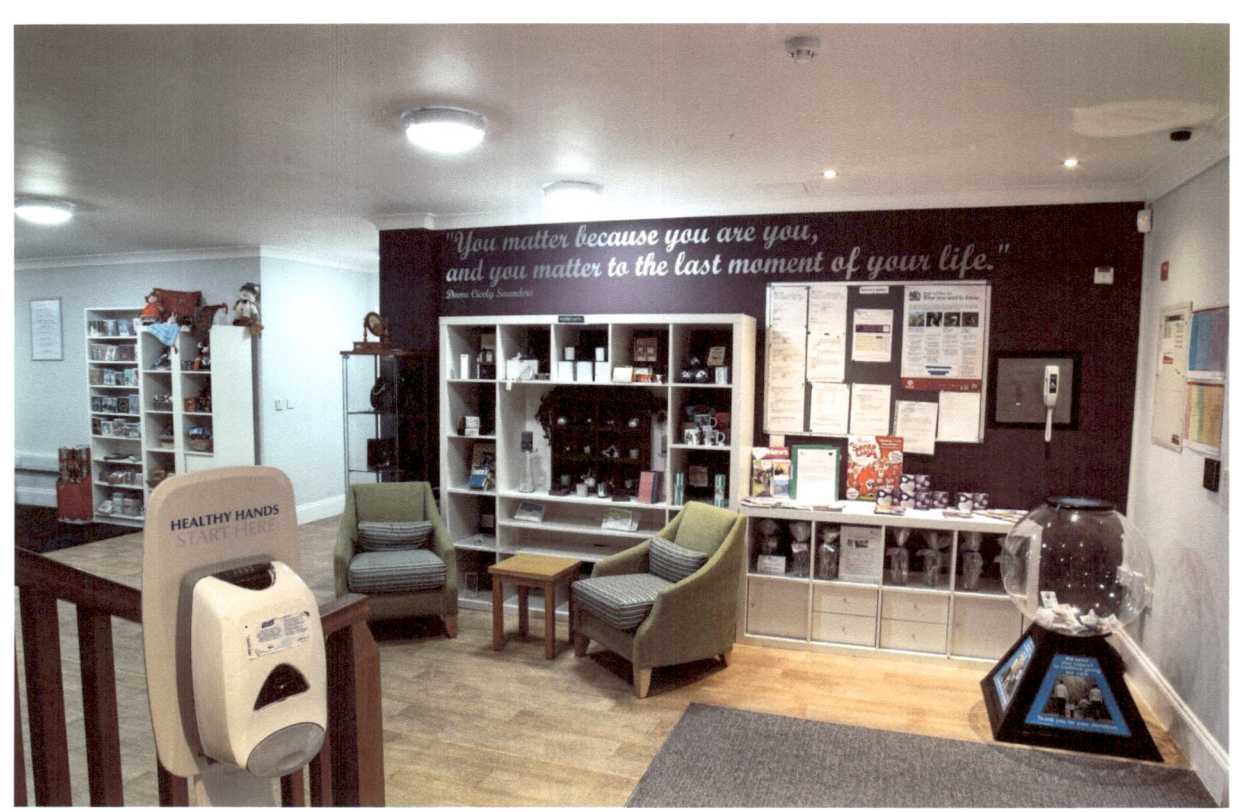

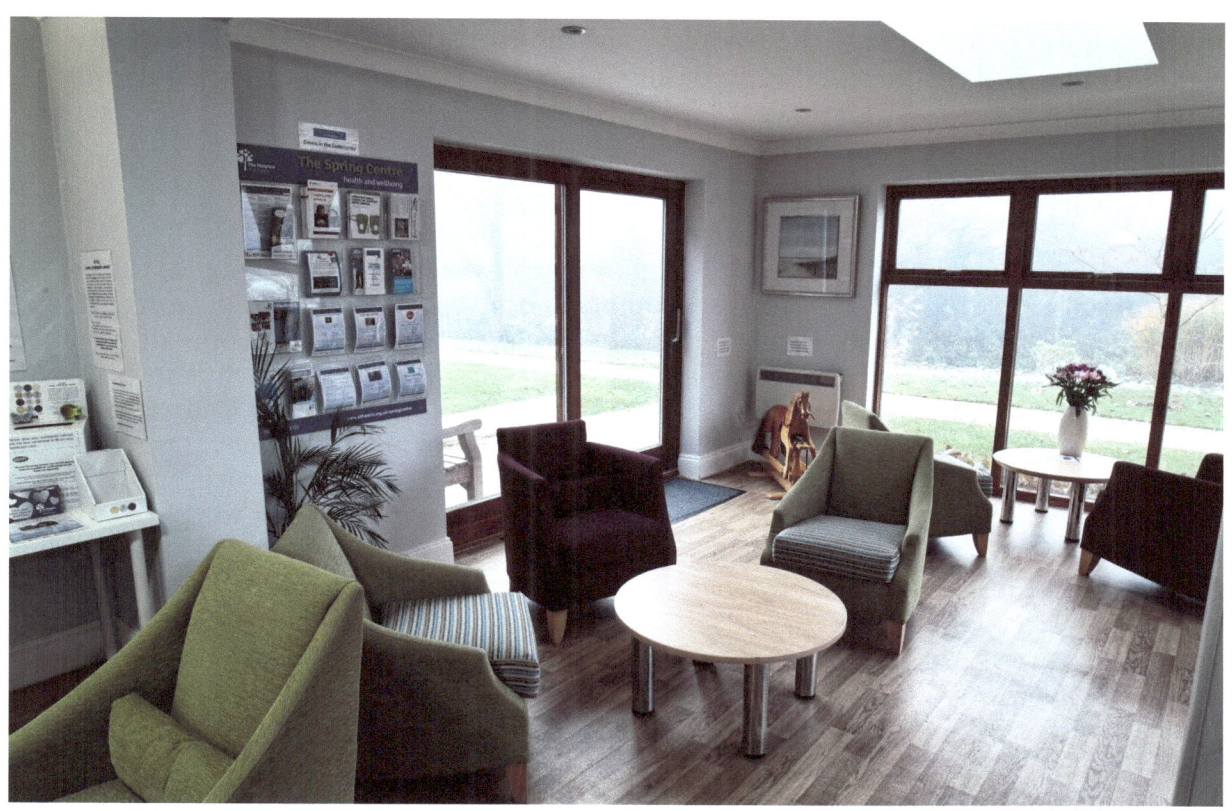

In The Spring Centre there is always something colourful around the corner and, often, you are greeted by someone special. The waiting area within The Spring Centre reception is a lovely, relaxing place filled with light and calm, full of interesting things and providing a warm welcome to the Hospice. The rooms within The Spring Centre are bright and cheerful, with little things adding interest for visitors. Such rooms do much to lift the spirit for patients and their families.

"As soon as I arrived at The Hospice of St Francis, it was a relief to be in such a safe environment, surrounded by caring people. Nobody should find the word 'Hospice' frightening - it's quite the reverse and the whole atmosphere is one of positivity, encouragement and care. The medical side of things is always there, but in a way that supports and promotes wellbeing. In the health and wellbeing Spring Centre, across the other side of the Hospice from the Inpatient Unit, they run some excellent courses and classes and I was able to join in an Art Therapy group, which was great fun, making jewellery beads from paper - something I'd never done before. My zest for life diminished when I became poorly but the Hospice put me on the road to regaining my confidence and that has continued. My state of mind is the complete opposite to what it was. The Hospice is a place full of life as well as being a place where some people might choose to die, but the care it provides is tailored to what each individual person needs at whatever stage of their illness. It just takes away the stress and uncertainty and supports families so well too, taking away the worry from them. I don't know how I would have coped without it."

Cheryl, patient

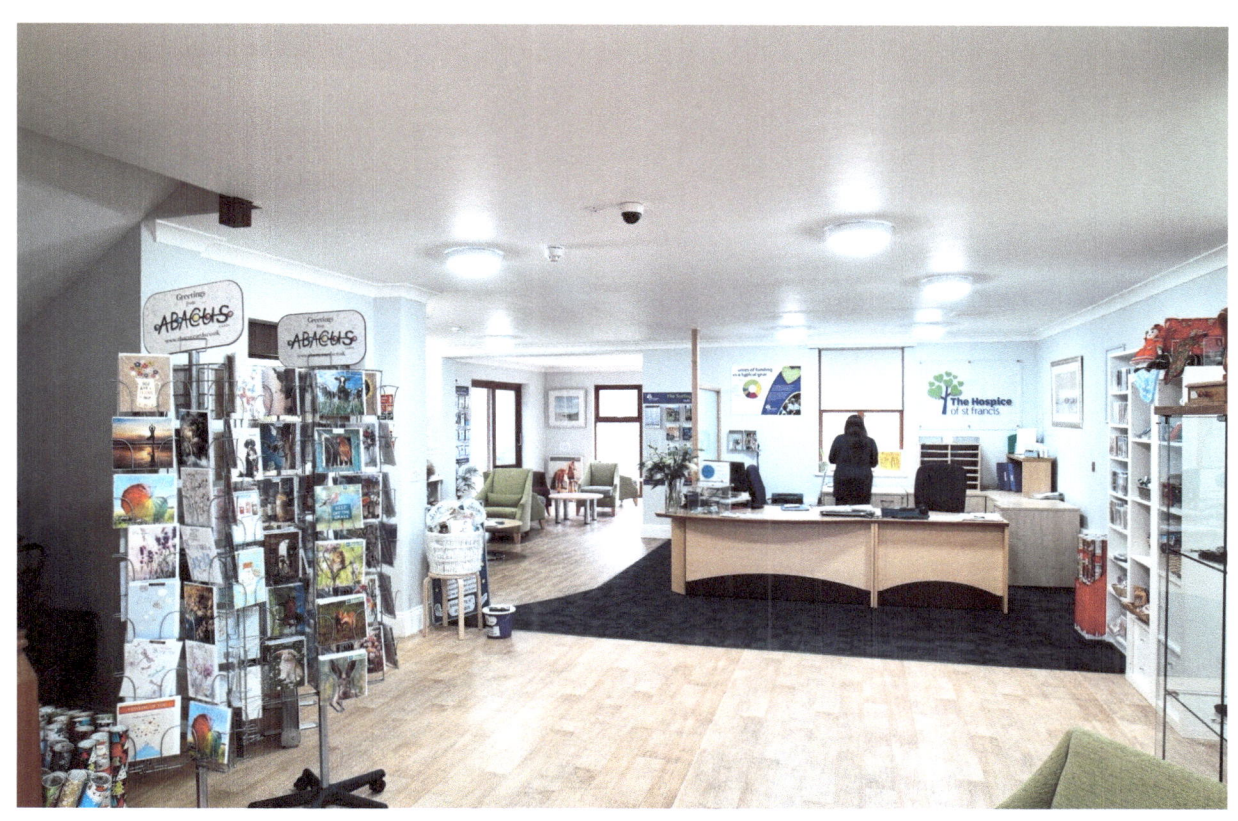

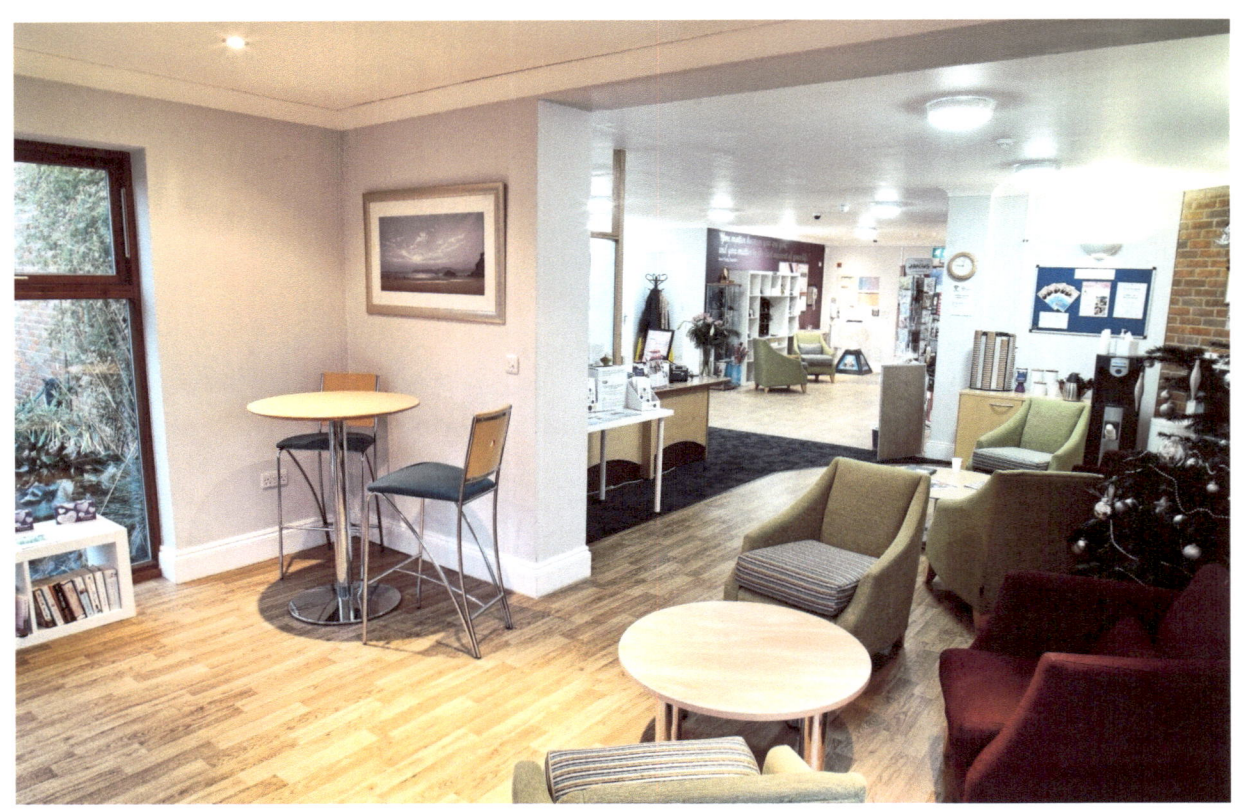

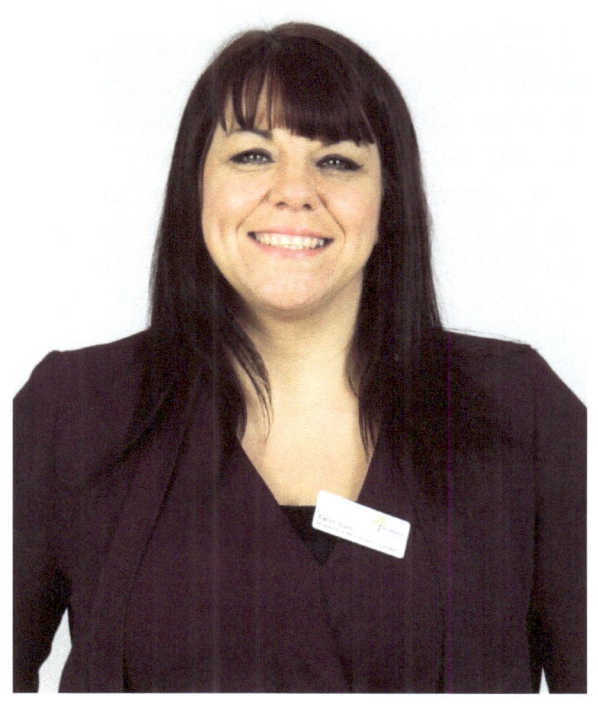

Karen
Reception and Office Services Coordinator

"I first had connections with the Hospice on a personal level and we could not have asked for any more support than what was offered. The help we had from the Children's Services team was invaluable at such a dark and scary time. I now feel so very lucky to be working here and when I see what people go through on a daily basis at the Hospice. It brings me great comfort, knowing that they are having the best help that they possibly can by people who are passionate about what they do and people who genuinely care. There is probably not a day I do not take something away with me - sometimes sad, but more often I take away something warm and there is always laughter in the day. The Hospice is a very special place."

The Spring Centre is a place like no other. It is a resource, a place, a community, a sanctuary, and more. Offering integrated and holistic support for those who have recently faced a diagnosis, who are living with, or are recovering from a significant illness, and for those who care for them, The Spring Centre gathers in all aspects of life - physical, mental, emotional, spiritual, practical - and focuses on the person at the centre of them all. The combination of specialist medical and nursing assessment with complementary and creative therapies, psychological support, practical advice - all in a place to learn, talk and share - makes The Spring Centre unique and invaluable for those who go there.

"I was in hospital for a week and when I was back home again, all I could concentrate on was recovering physically from a very painful and debilitating procedure. It took up all my energy during the first couple of months. Emotionally however, I was still in a state of shock. I really needed to talk to someone. I was lying awake at night, feeling anxious, afraid that the cancer might come back, and afraid of having to cope long-term with something so debilitating. In April 2014, my GP referred me to the Hospice's Spring Centre health and wellbeing hub as an outpatient. In essence, Julie (a Clinical Specialist Nurse, who saw me at The Spring Centre) has got me back to my normal positive self and brought me to a place where I can accept that things happen, and you just have to deal with them and move on. We can worry all we like about what's happened or what may happen, but what we should be focusing on is life in the here and now. I had no idea the Hospice could help someone like me and that its help could make such a valuable difference to my recovery. I honestly thought it was a place where people come to die and to find out that it's not has been a big surprise. It's a beautiful calming environment, everyone greets you with a smile, the receptionist remembers your name and you just feel so welcome. The whole experience has been really, really positive. I feel very lucky that it's been here for me and for that I'm really grateful."

Julia, outpatient

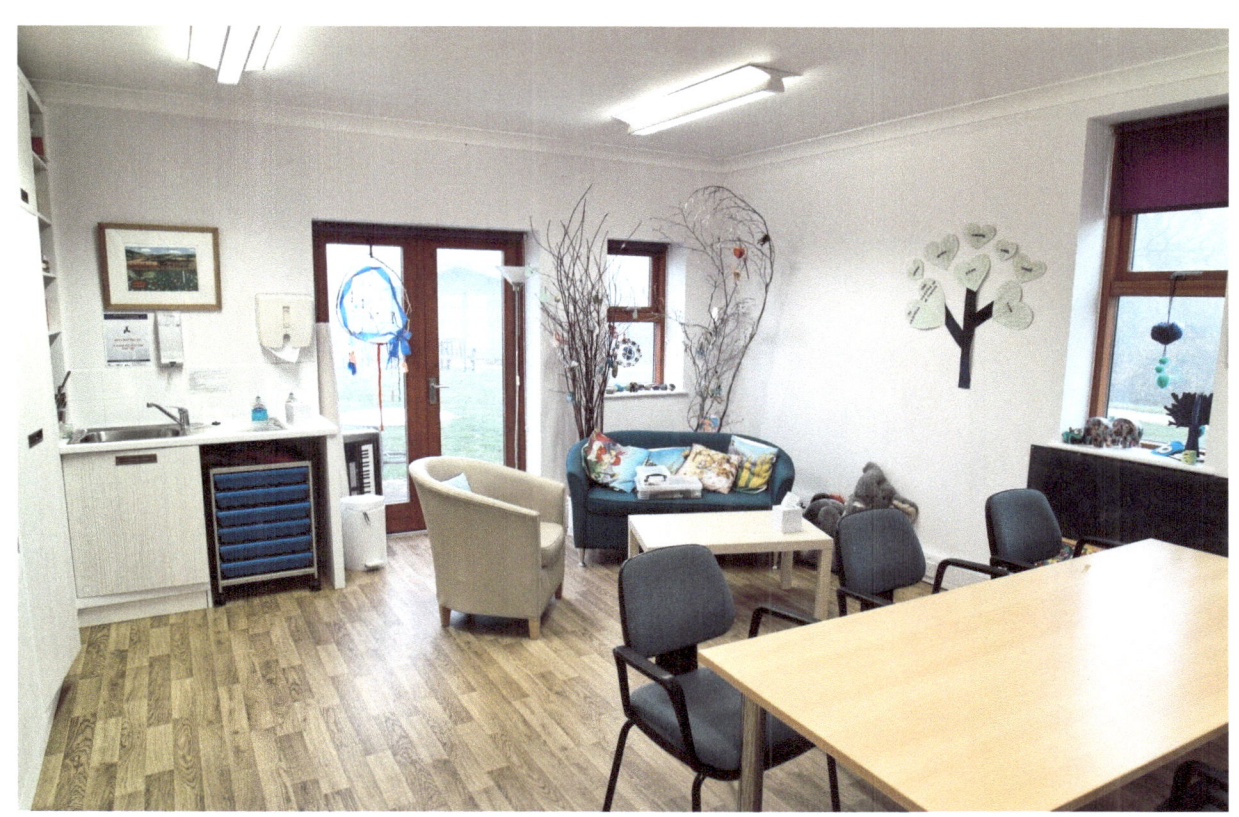

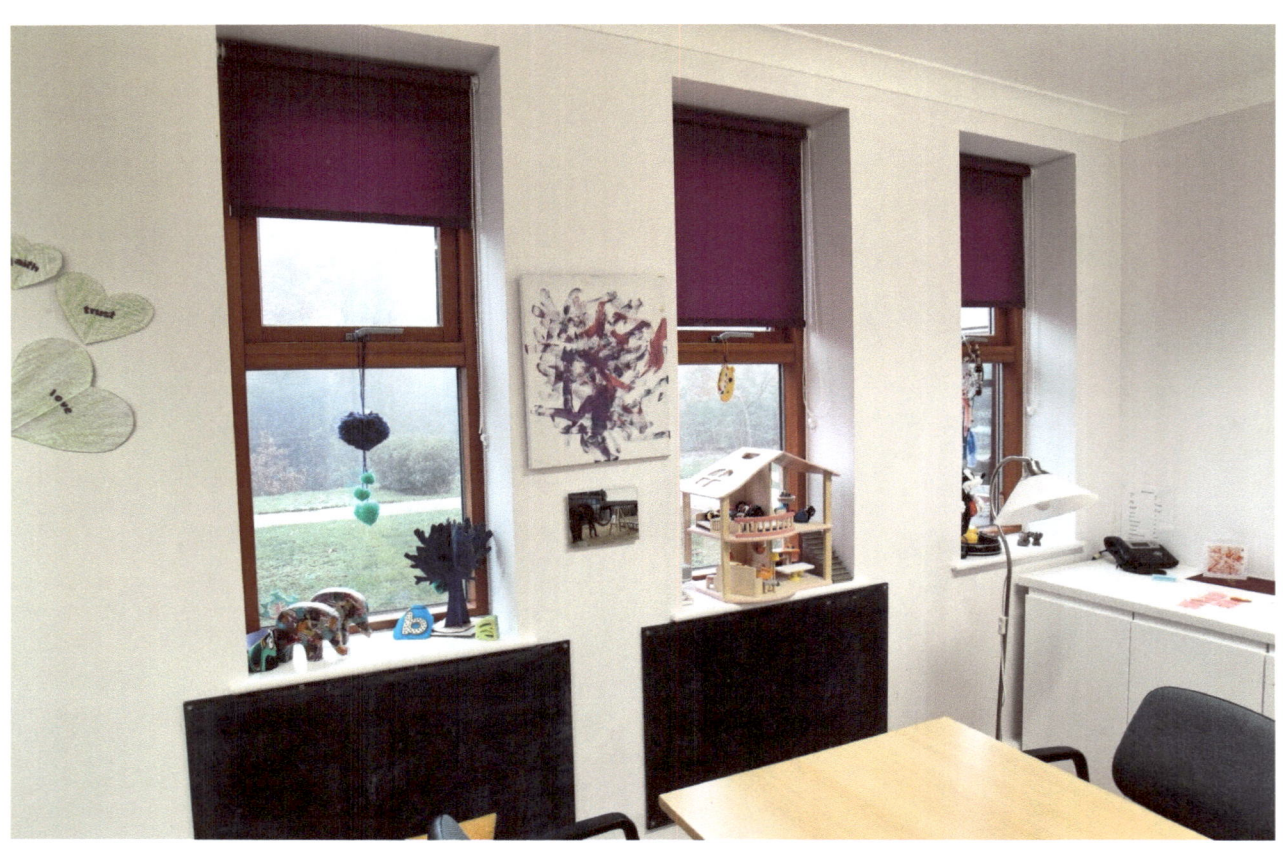

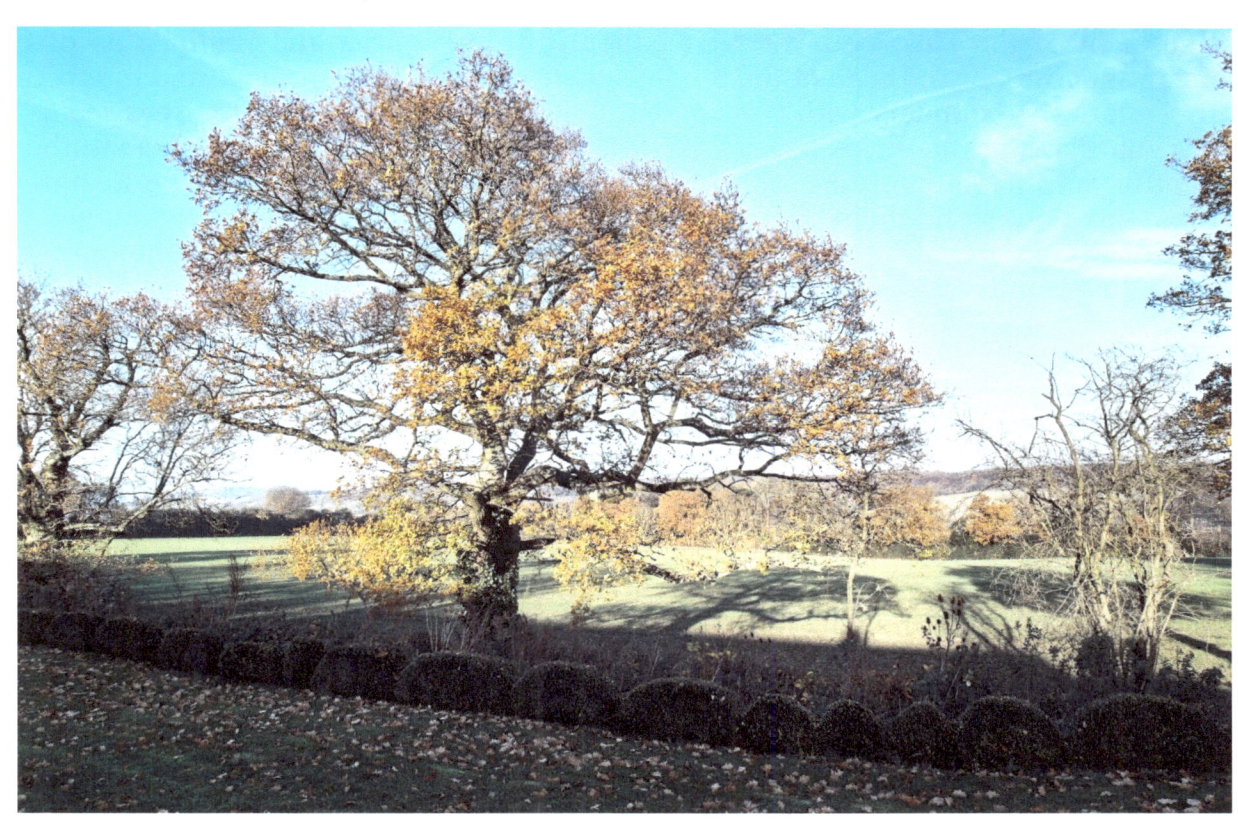

Looking out across the fields from the windows and gardens, one might easily forget that we are situated in the busy market town of Berkhamsted. There are many beautiful trees within sight of the Hospice. Just seeing them lifts the spirits and reminds us of the wonder of nature. At the edge of the immediate grounds a blaze of colour and interesting shrubs mark the boundary with the surrounding fields, and the beautiful trees seems to act as guardians for the fields beyond. No artist's palette could produce such a swathe of delightful hues in the morning sun. Mother Nature has all the best colours. Evergreen shrubs and flowers brighten the view as we gaze out across the fields adjoining the Hospice grounds. On the woodland path, occasionally, a vista opens out onto the surrounding countryside.

"I really hadn't wanted to leave my home and I was really anxious about handing over my care. The nurses couldn't have been kinder though, telling me not to worry and explaining that the Hospice wasn't just a place where people come to die but somewhere you leave and come back to again when you need it. Just those few words really helped calm and reassure me, enabling me to start processing what I knew and understand more about what was going on in my body. The nurses were so attentive and so many doctors came to see me, listening and talking me through my options and always making sure that my husband was included. Nothing was too much trouble. Rob and I both knew I was in the right place and we'll never forget that feeling of relief. The minute we crossed the threshold, it was like being cuddled - and that feeling of being hugged has never gone away. They pampered me and made me feel special but the biggest thing they gave me was my independence and the confidence to know I could go home.

Charlie, patient

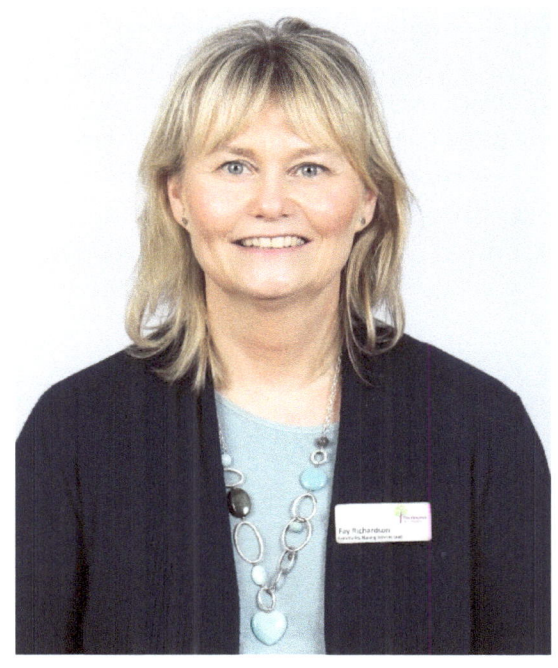

Fay
Community Nursing Services Lead

"I am lucky enough to be part of The Hospice of St Francis as the Nursing lead for the Community Team. The team has grown in capacity and is therefore able to see more people with life-limiting illness at various stages of their illness and support their families. This energetic, enthusiastic team embraces change and development, now seeing more outpatients in The Spring Centre and working closely with other health care providers. This is such a rewarding role, knowing we help so many patients and their families through the shock of diagnosis of a life-limiting illness and supporting them throughout their ongoing journey, be that at diagnosis or at end of life. I thrive on the challenges of leading such a compassionate, caring, driven and adaptable team, providing excellent care and service to all we meet."

The Hospice reaches beyond its own walls in so many ways, not least of which is through the work of the Community Team. Most patients would prefer to be at home, and Hospice doctors, nurses, therapists and members of the supportive care team - as well as committed volunteers - will take the same professionalism, compassion and respect out into the community. There's always the phone too, with a friendly voice and a listening ear there to offer help and support - be that physical, emotional, or practical. How important it is to have a team that knows what you need and, even more importantly, who you are - and is there, by your side, when you need them.

"Speaking to the Hospice is the best thing I've ever done. I've had more help from the Hospice than anyone – they've been absolutely brilliant and Louise, my community nurse, has been a godsend. They're always at the end of the phone if I need them and if I'm feeling sorry for myself, I'll speak to Louise and she'll get me out of it."

Bill, patient

"I realise now I had no idea what hospices do. They're about support, help, caring and sharing, and The Hospice of St Francis has been the support structure that's helped me through the most difficult time of my life. I live alone so Liz, my community nurse, has been the family I don't have on the doorstep. She's been amazing."

Matt, patient

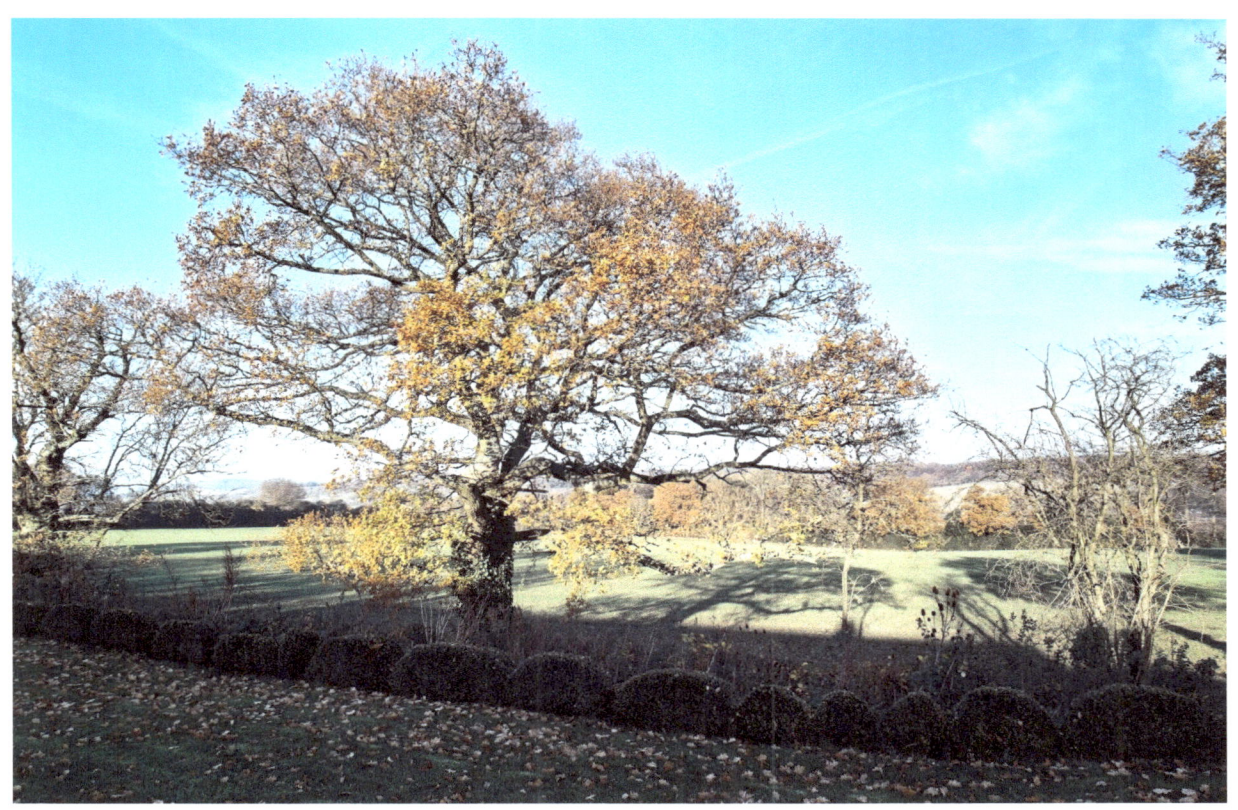

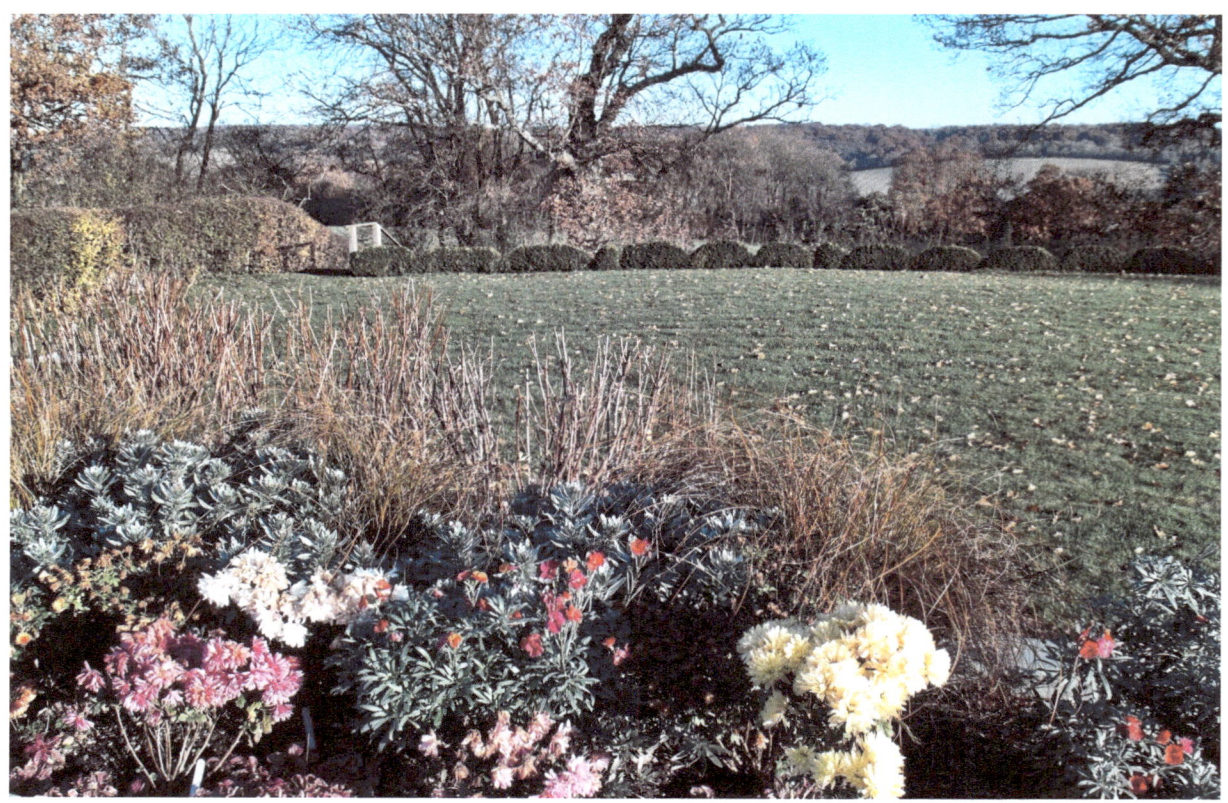

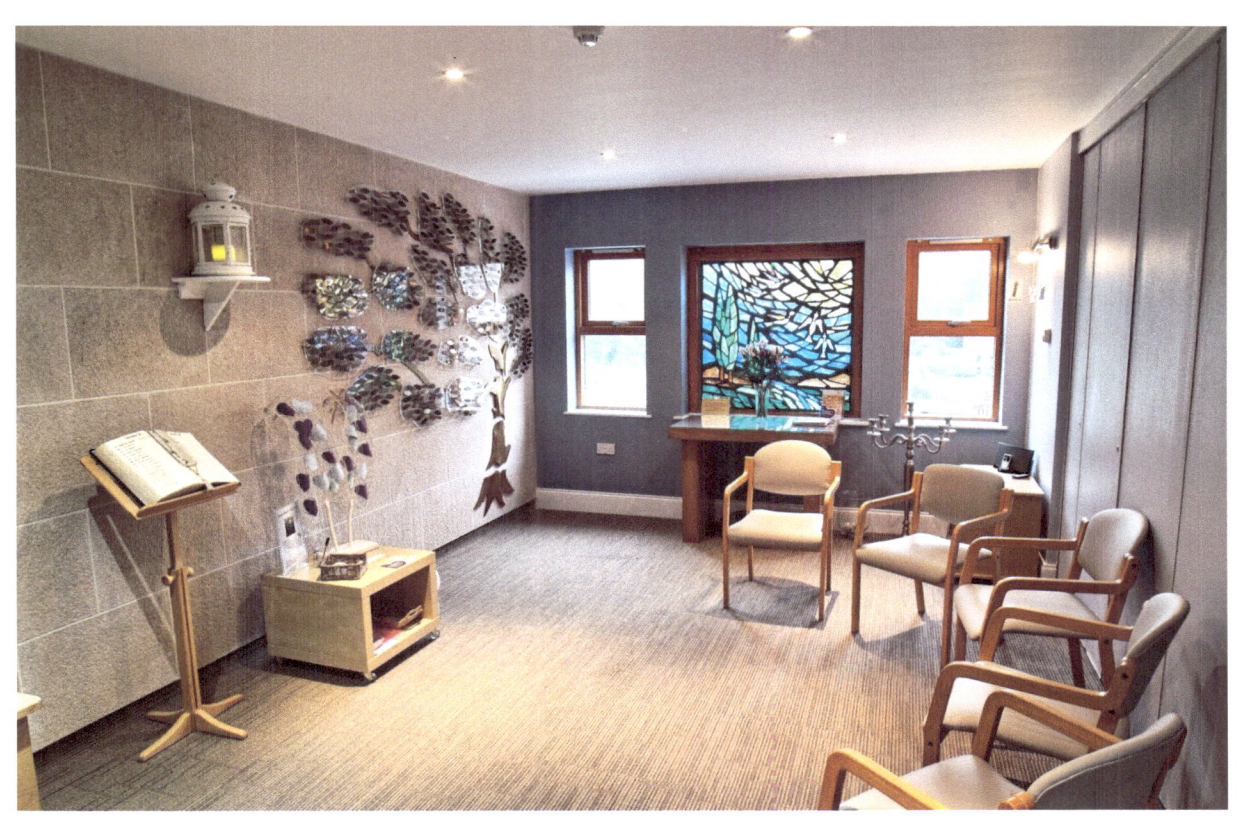

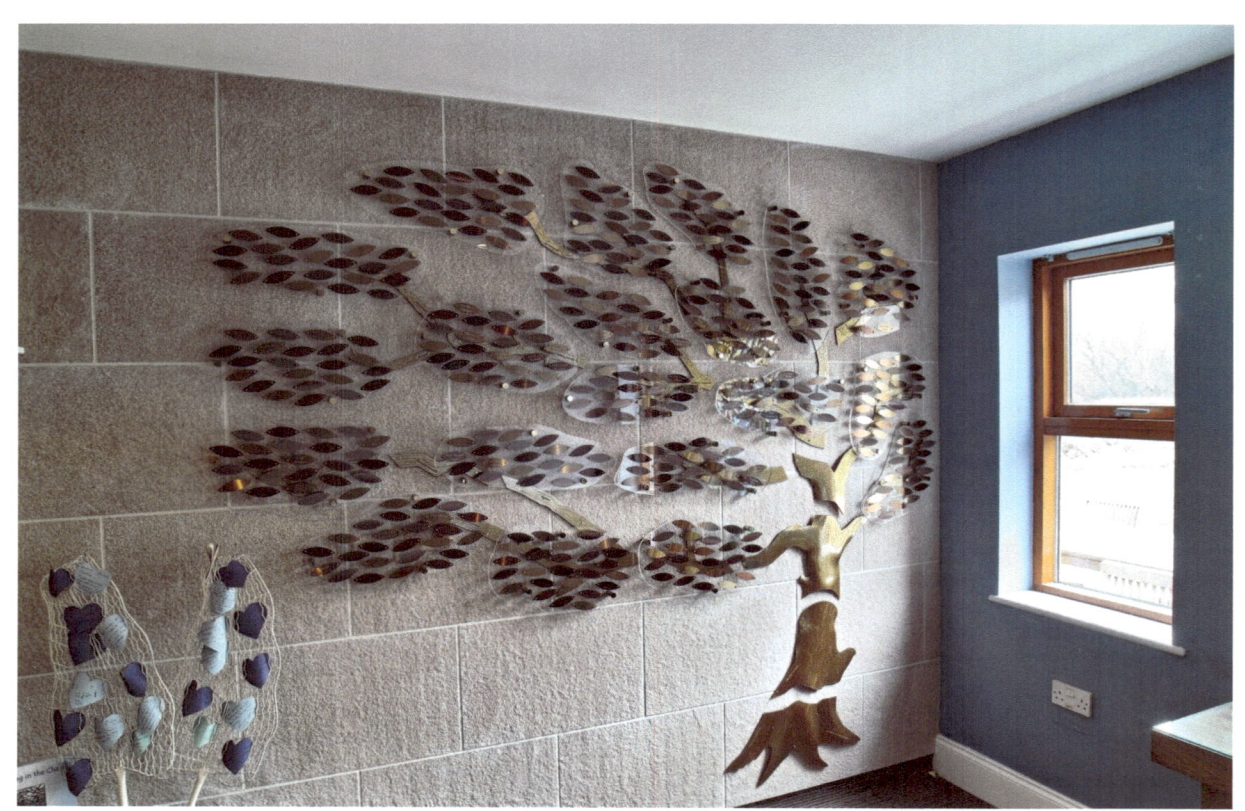

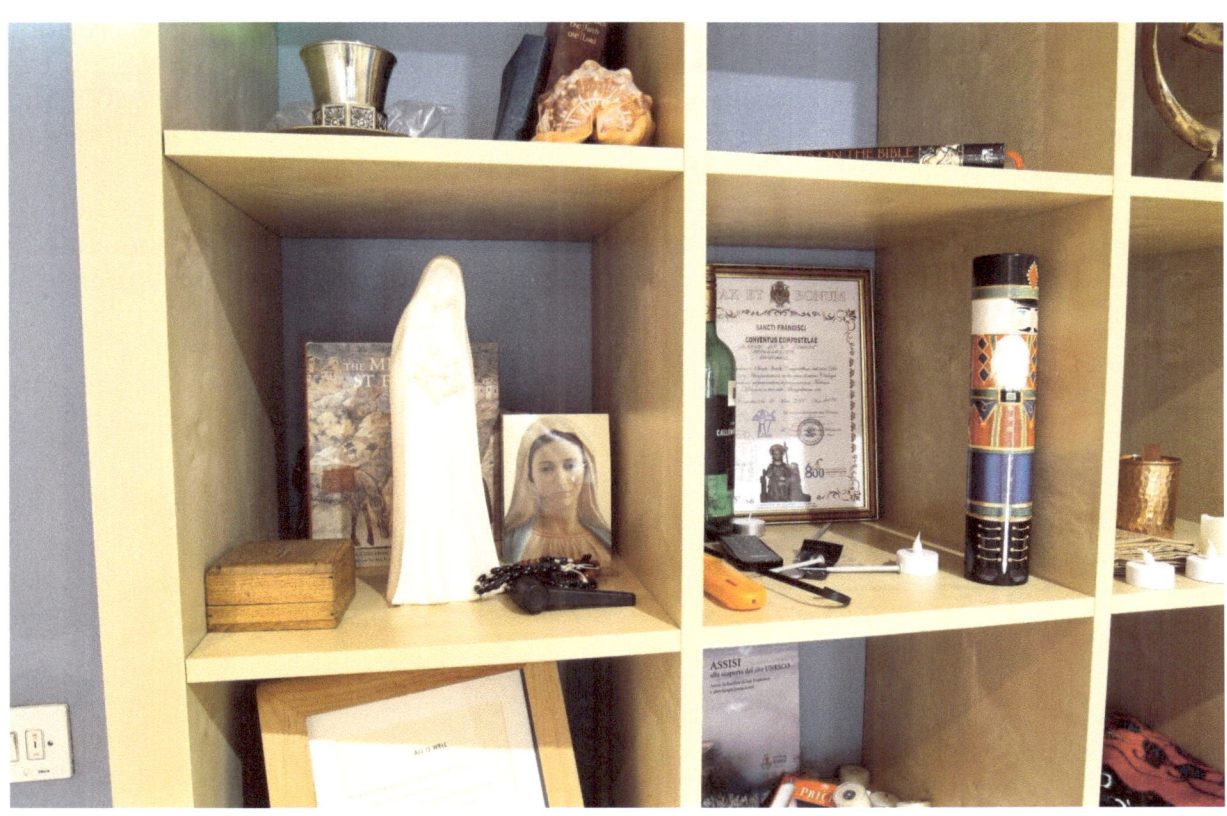

The beautiful little Chapel exudes peace and calm and yet is also uplifting with its lovely stained glass window and warm colours. The Memory Tree within the Chapel is a lovely idea and beautifully executed. Every day, the morning sun illuminates those precious memories. There is a quiet corner of the Chapel where one may sit and reflect. On the shelves are to be found a variety of delightful little statues and objects to discover and give pleasure. The Chapel holds the Book of Remembrance, too, where the names of many friends who have passed through the Hospice, will always be remembered.

"The Hospice gives me peace of mind. I know I have somewhere to go to and someone to talk to when I need help. The Hospice has been a lifeline to me and I can't recommend it highly enough to anyone who needs support."

Frank, patient

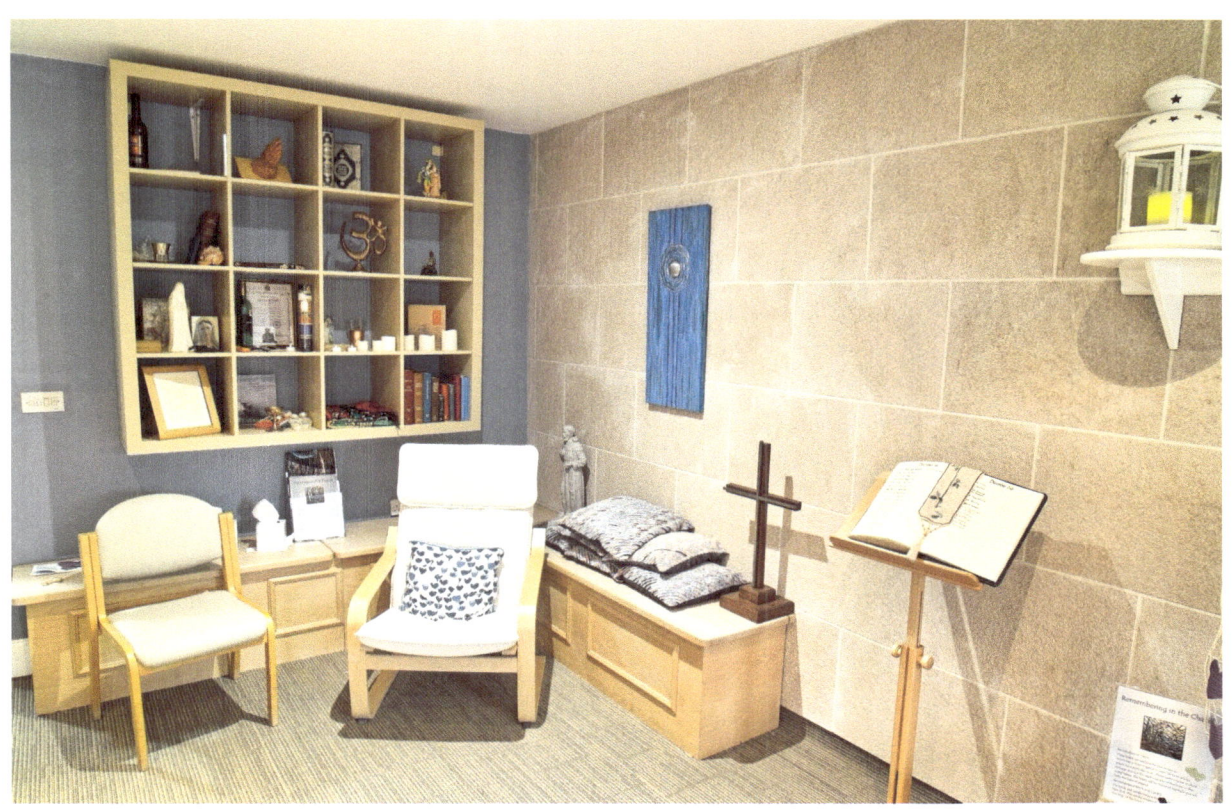

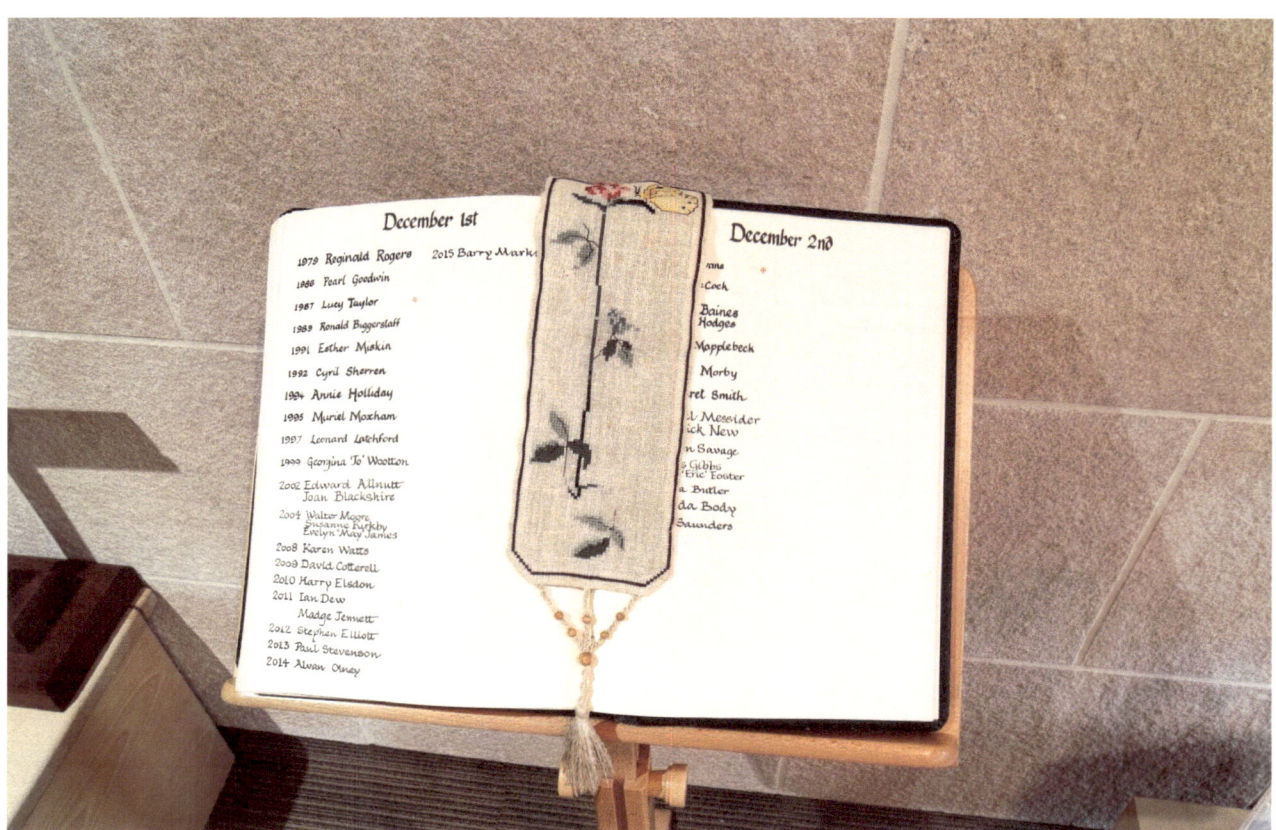

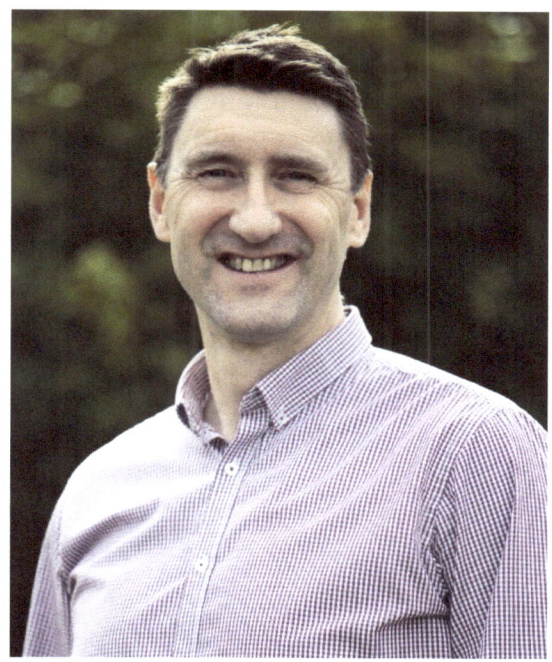

Ray
Chaplain

"When people hear what I do their initial reaction is often, 'that must be so depressing'. Actually, although there are obviously some very sad situations, my job at the Hospice is *life-affirming*. Being able to get to know patients and families at such a significant time is a real privilege and I get immense satisfaction from it. At The Hospice of St Francis, we want people to feel free to express their spirituality or practise their religion in their own way - or not at all. Spiritual care is about finding out what's important to a person, ensuring we are treating them as an individual and offering a listening ear. Our Chapel has been set aside as a restful space, providing a quiet place for reflection and remembrance for people from various faith backgrounds and none. We hope that an atheist or agnostic will feel just as much at home in the space as a religious person."

In the peace of the Chapel, everyone can bring their faith - or lack thereof, their doubts, their fears, their hopes. Patients, families, staff and volunteers can all find a quiet space there. The Remembrance Book honours the memory of all who have passed on under the care of the Hospice, listing the names in beautiful calligraphy. On the wall, the Memory Tree's hundreds of leaves capture the light as it glints on the names inscribed there. The stunning stained-glass window, designed and made by French artist Jaques Loire, is a reminder of the building in which the Hospice found its first home - the convent on Shrublands Road.

"Just days after he was admitted, Paul passed away peacefully with me by his side. The Hospice Chaplain said the most beautiful prayer, which ended with the words, 'Go on your travels my friend, be safe', and I saw Paul relax as though he realised it was okay now for him to go."

Eleanor, family member

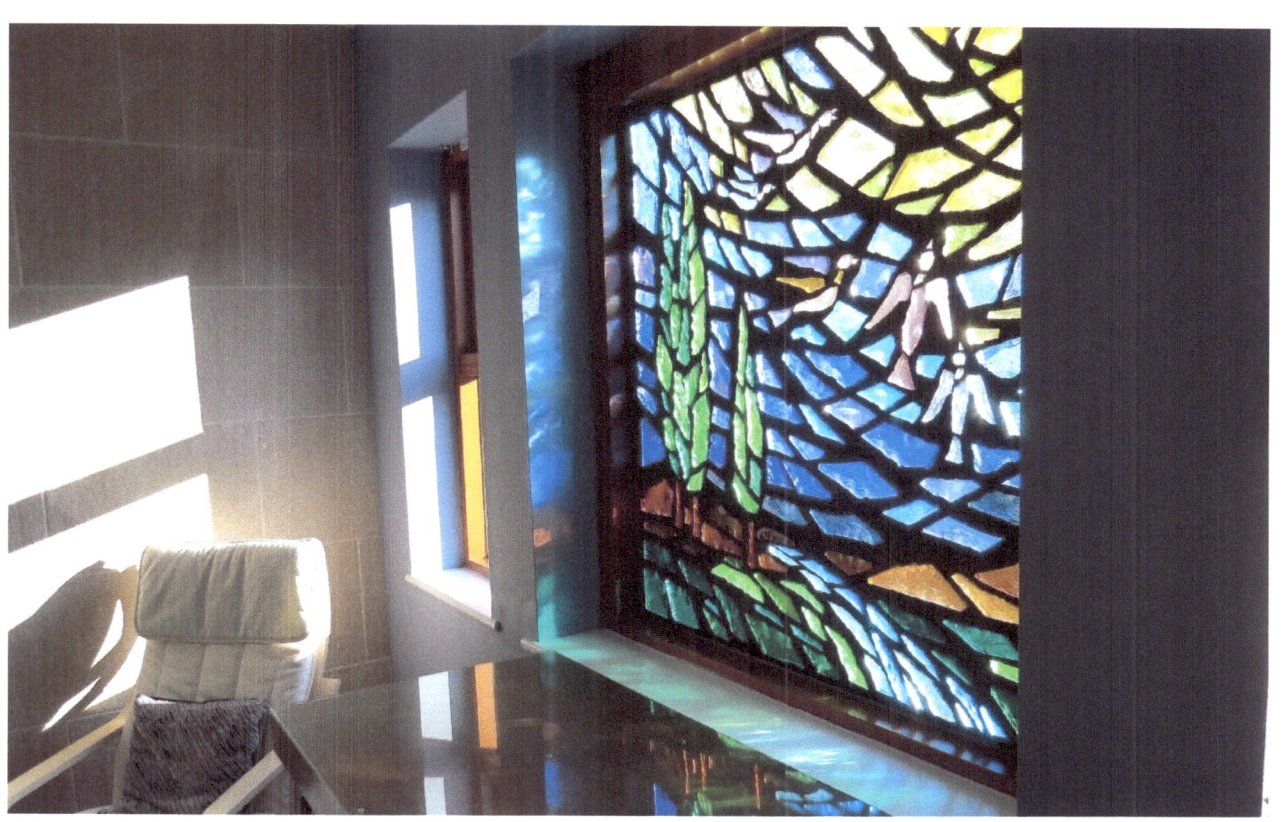

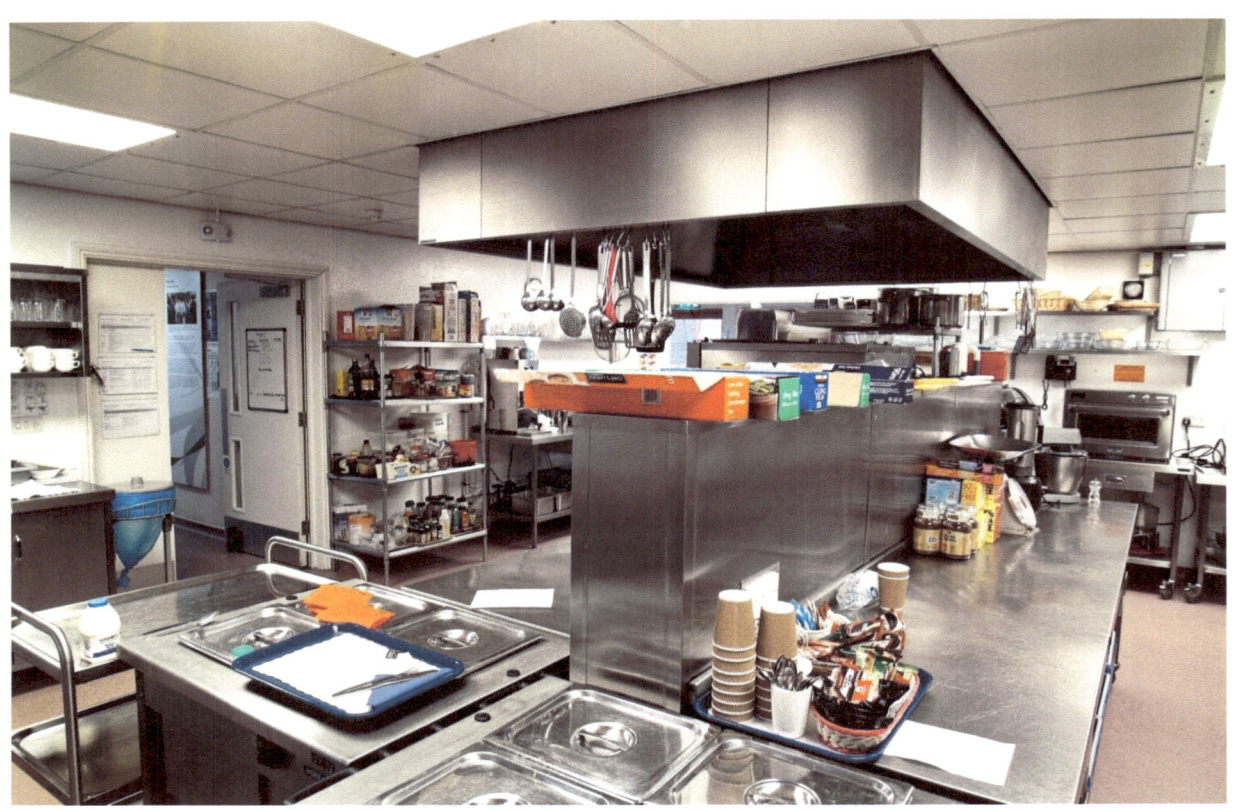

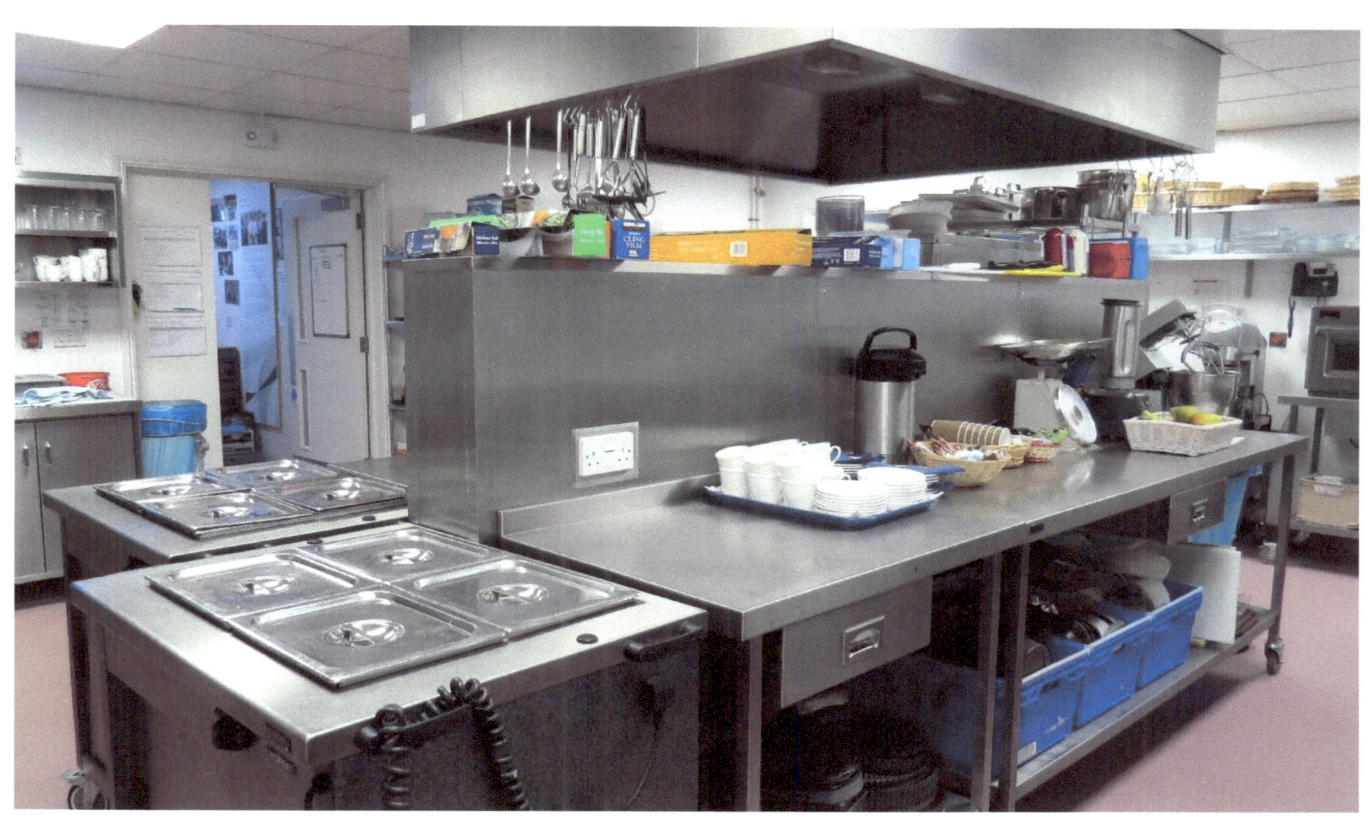

The magnificent kitchen area, at the heart of the Hospice, is where a wide selection of nutritious meals are prepared for patients. The serving hatch opens in welcome from the bistro onto the kitchen area. Patients and visitors may also make themselves a nice cup of tea here. Good food, carefully and lovingly prepared, is at the centre of the Hospice's philosophy of total care. A freshly prepared meal - or even a simple smoothie to tempt an ailing appetite - can make all the difference, strengthening body and mind.

"Linda and I both knew that the Hospice was the best place for her to be. The level of support she'd received for her symptom control had given her great confidence in the Hospice and the staff, and she felt safe and very relieved that it had lifted a great part of the burden of care from me. In one word, the care and support was inspiring - the meticulous attention to detail, the reassurance, the encouragement, the comfort, the time. Nothing was too much trouble. On Christmas Day, they prepared a full Christmas dinner, with crackers and all the trimmings, for us and we ate it together. It's a lovely positive memory. Linda's first question was 'But who's going to look after Brian?' and the Medical Director told her: 'We will.' You can become very isolated and cut off from the world. But thanks to Cooking with Chris, here I was, back socialising with people and sitting around a table with people who wouldn't ask questions about my problems and knew what I was going through. It was just what I needed. It seems like only yesterday that she'd be asking me to cook if we had friends coming round for dinner. I happily used to do it – but thanks to the Hospice and Cooking with Chris, the choice today is a bit more varied and of that, I know Linda would have been proud. I was and still am overwhelmed by the way the Hospice's care surrounded, enfolded and supported my Linda, myself and my family both during her illness and afterwards. There were not enough words at the time. There are still not enough..."

Brian, family member and volunteer

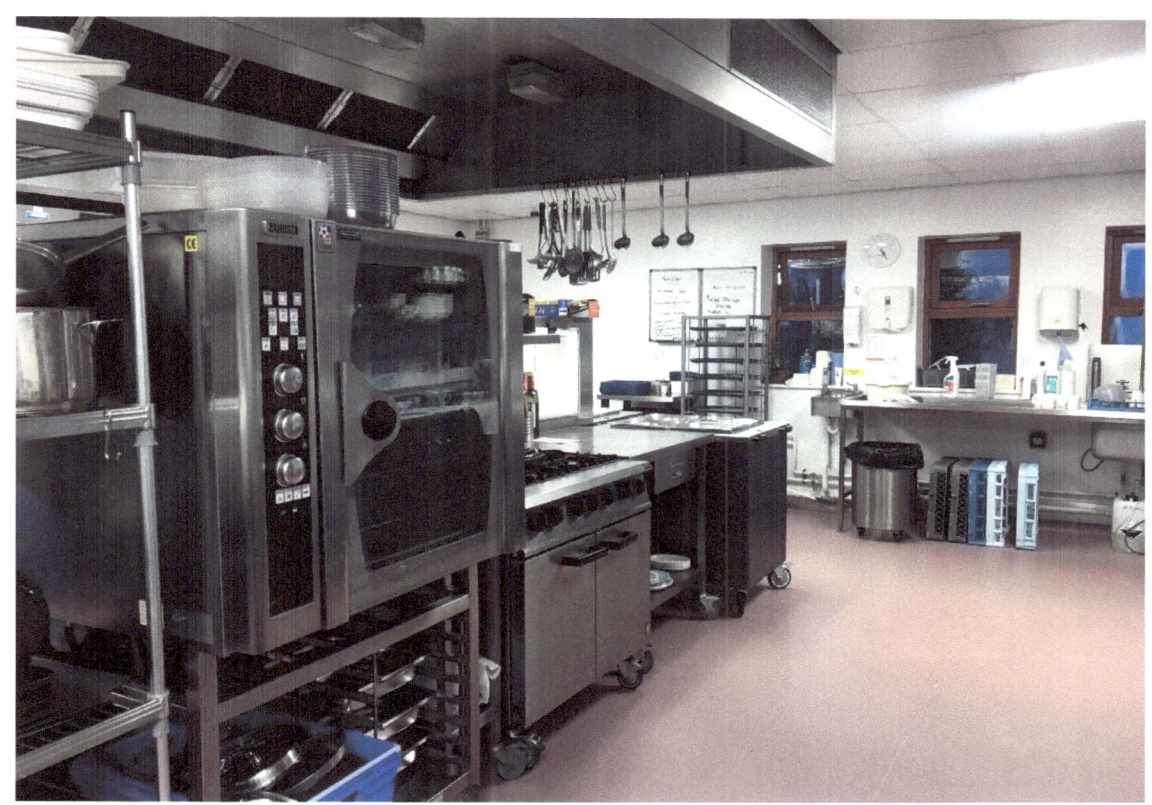

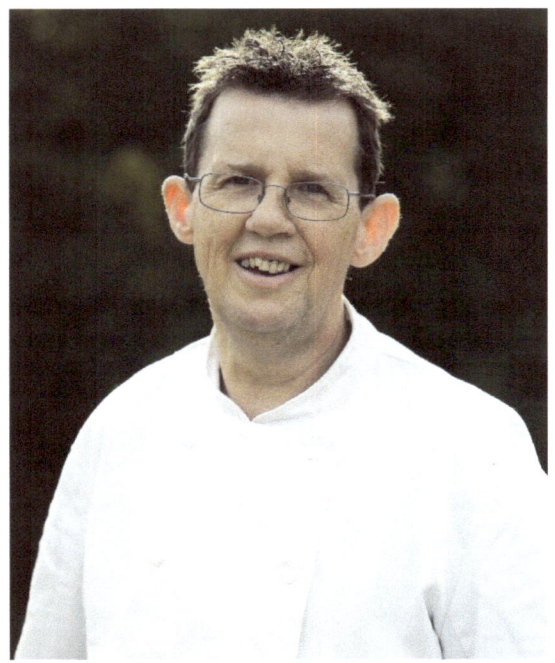

Chris
Catering Manager

"I always say food is love. Food is an opportunity to bring patients and families together in the moment, whether it's for a Sunday lunch, a birthday celebration or a special anniversary. On a day to day level here at the Hospice, it's also something that patients can control in terms of what they like, how they like it cooked, how big or small a portion they want and how it's presented. My whole team and I take great pride in every plate we send out because sometimes we only have one chance to get it right. I had a note from a patient just this morning to say how much she'd enjoyed her mushrooms on toast for breakfast – it's at times like that that I feel I'm doing my job right!"

Right at the heart of the Hospice is the kitchen - just as in any loving home. The attention to detail and to good home-cooked food is central to the way patients and their families are taken care of here. Bringing back appetites that have been long lost, putting together family dinners with familiar flavours, relieving the anxiety that can surround food - the team in the kitchen meet families, talk to patients, discover tastes and preferences, choices and restrictions, and work to restore the joy that sharing food together can bring as well as the peace of mind and strength of body that eating well can provide.

"After mum was sent home from hospital, as a family we were really struggling. Not only had the diagnosis come out of the blue, we were now left in a position where our mother was in constant pain and needed specialist care. Our GP was absolutely amazing. He knew that The Hospice of St Francis would be exactly the right place for mum and give us the support we needed as a family. After just an hour in the Hospice we felt we could relax. The staff took care of mum's needs and we felt a weight had been lifted off our shoulders. Her old personality appeared again and she didn't feel or look ill. Dad was also well looked after and was able to sleep at the Hospice and the catering team, led by Head Chef, Chris Took, prepared hot comforting meals for both my parents. We were able to spend quality family time together rather than stressing about having to sort out mum's medical and care needs, which was a huge relief. As well as providing 24-hour care for mum, and supporting dad, the Hospice team arranged for Carey and me, to get married in the Hospice chapel. We'd been planning a wedding for the September of 2012 but wanted to bring it forward so mum could witness our special day. It took place on 5th July and was a lovely occasion and full of special memories for us and our three young children. Mum stayed at the Hospice for five days before she passed away on 8th July 2012, just seven weeks after diagnosis, at the age of 69. We'd never done anything for charity before but were blown away by the care she received and have been driven ever since to help raise money to fund the specialist end of life care the Hospice provides."

David, family member

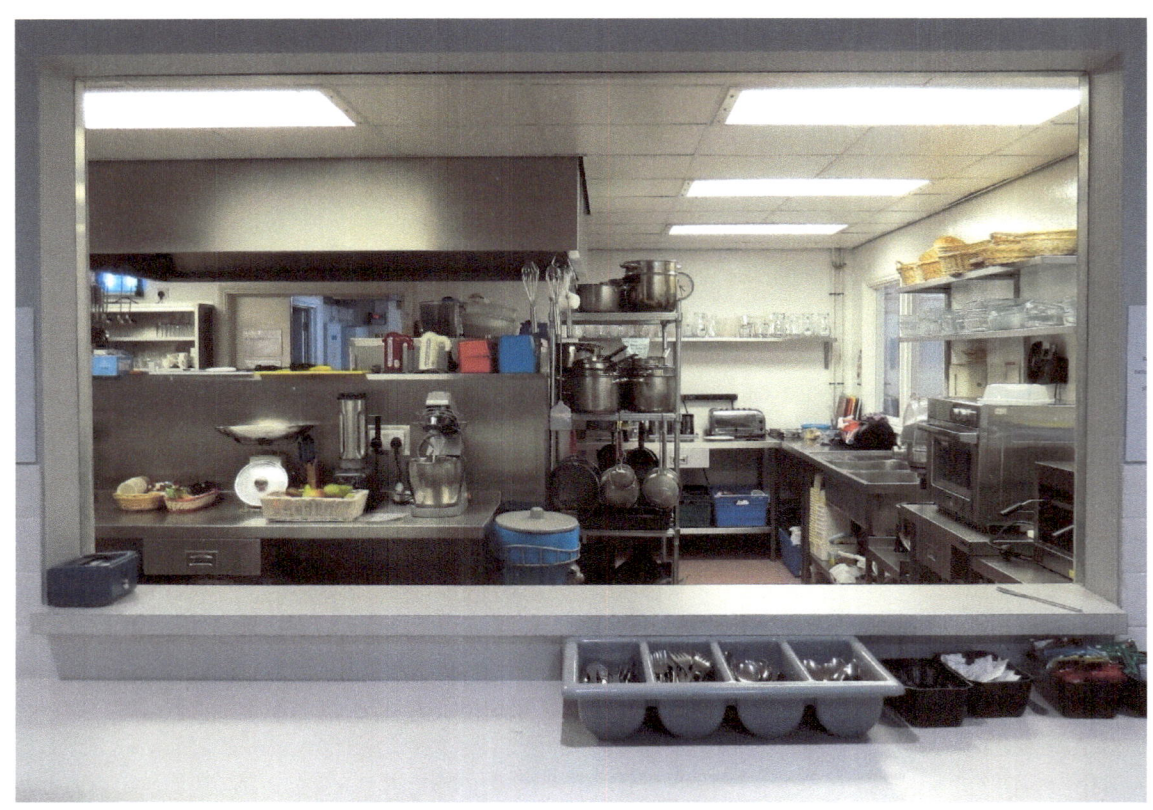

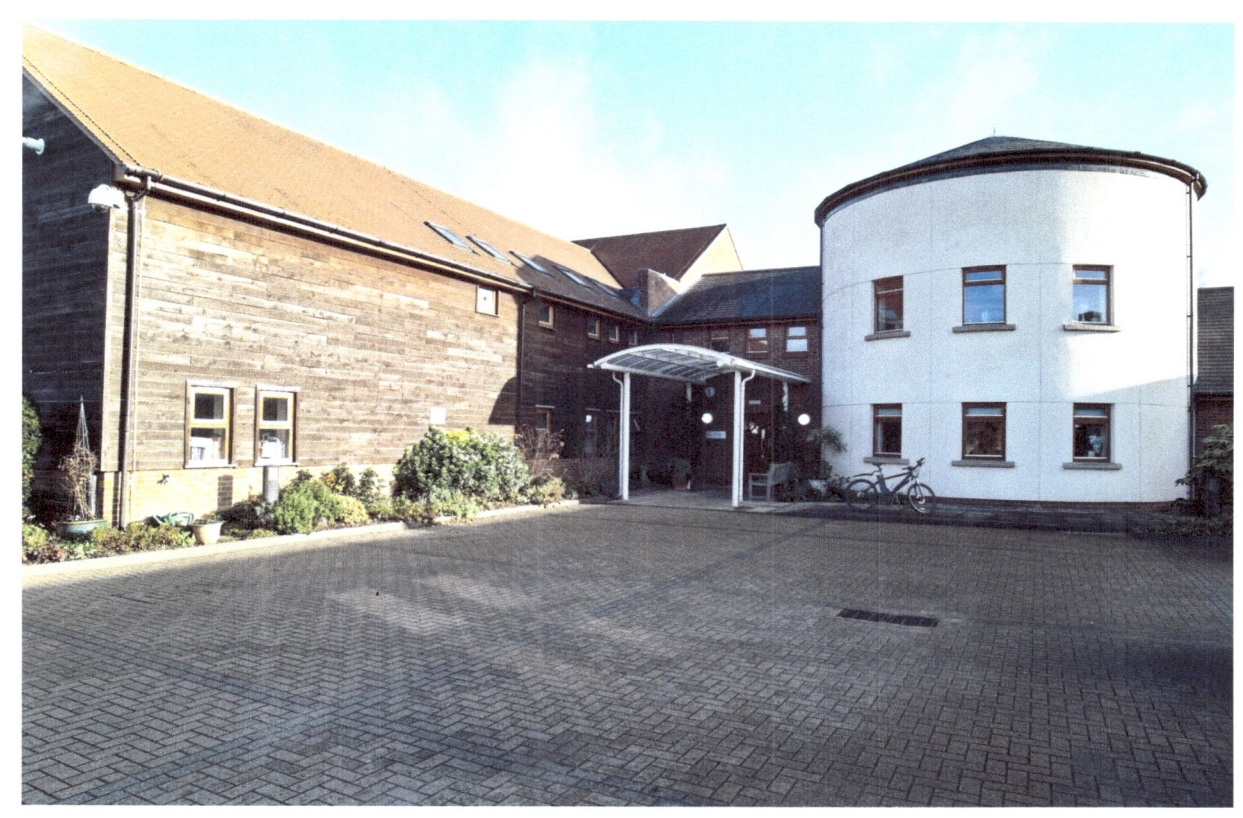

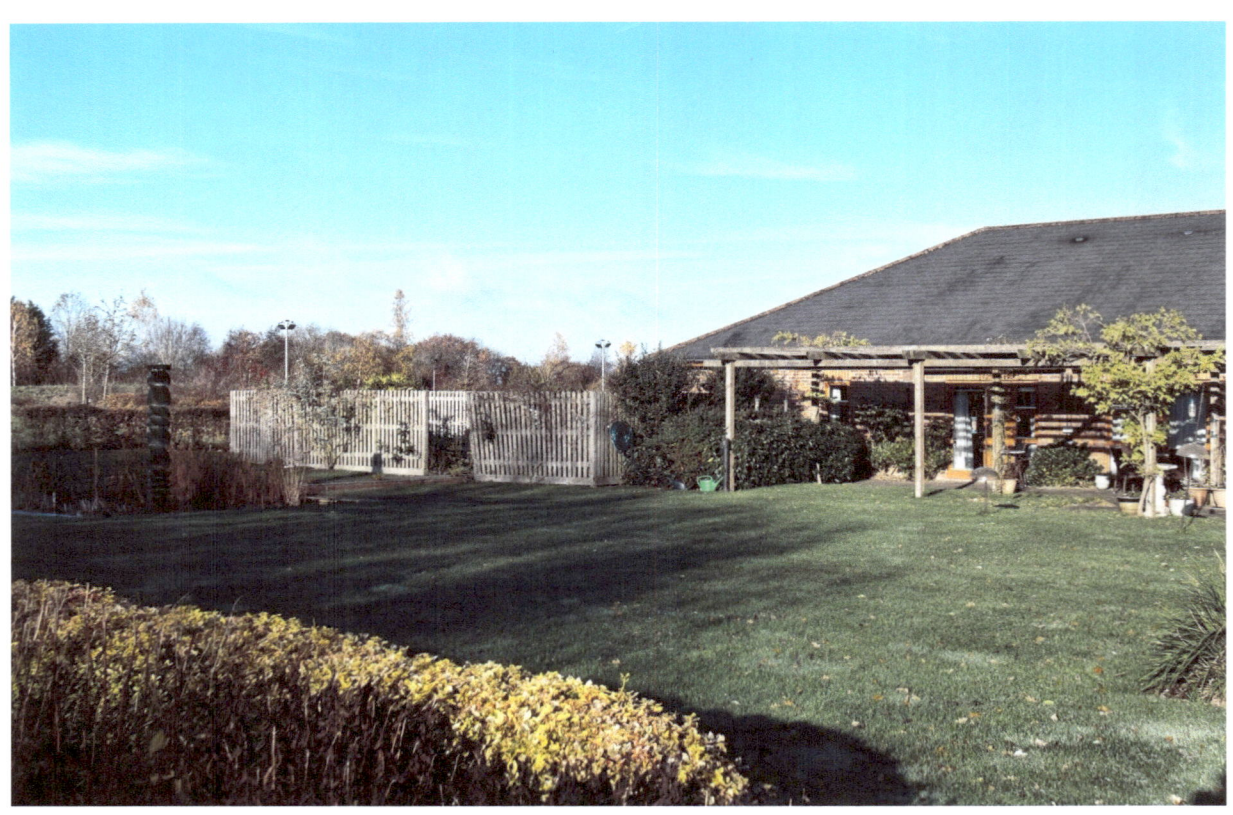

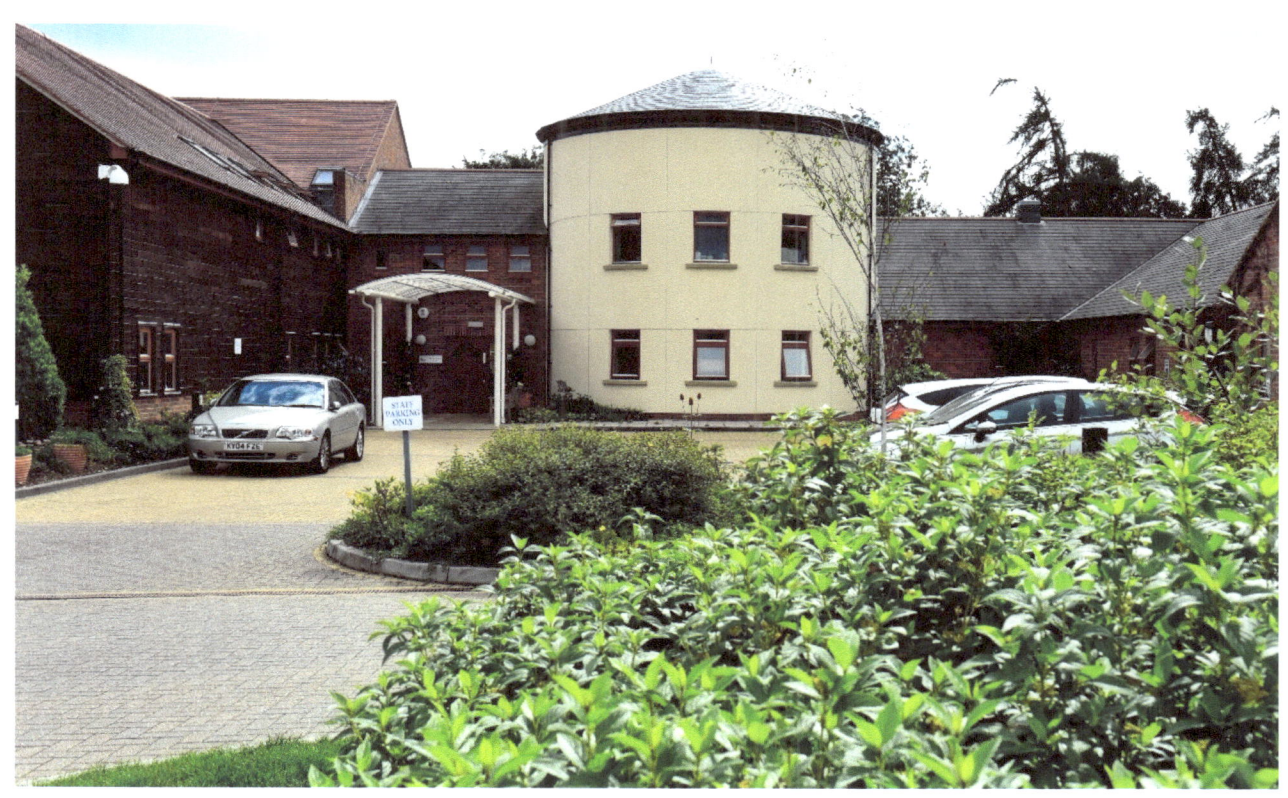

So many people have been grateful to walk through that door to the Inpatient Unit at The Hospice of St Francis. The entrance to the unit is both inviting and functional. Patients have a beautiful view of the grounds from their room, looking out across the lawn to the gardens and edge of the woodlands. All rooms have patio doors opening out onto the lawns. If the weather is agreeable, patients may like to sit outside for a while, or even lie outside in their bed. Inside the common lounge area there are comfortable chairs and a large television for those who like to watch.

"Being a milkman means I meet hundreds of people from all walks of life, which helps me chat to anyone on the Inpatient Unit. I hope that by greeting everyone with a friendly smile or a kind word, I can help others to cope with their situation."

Mick, volunteer

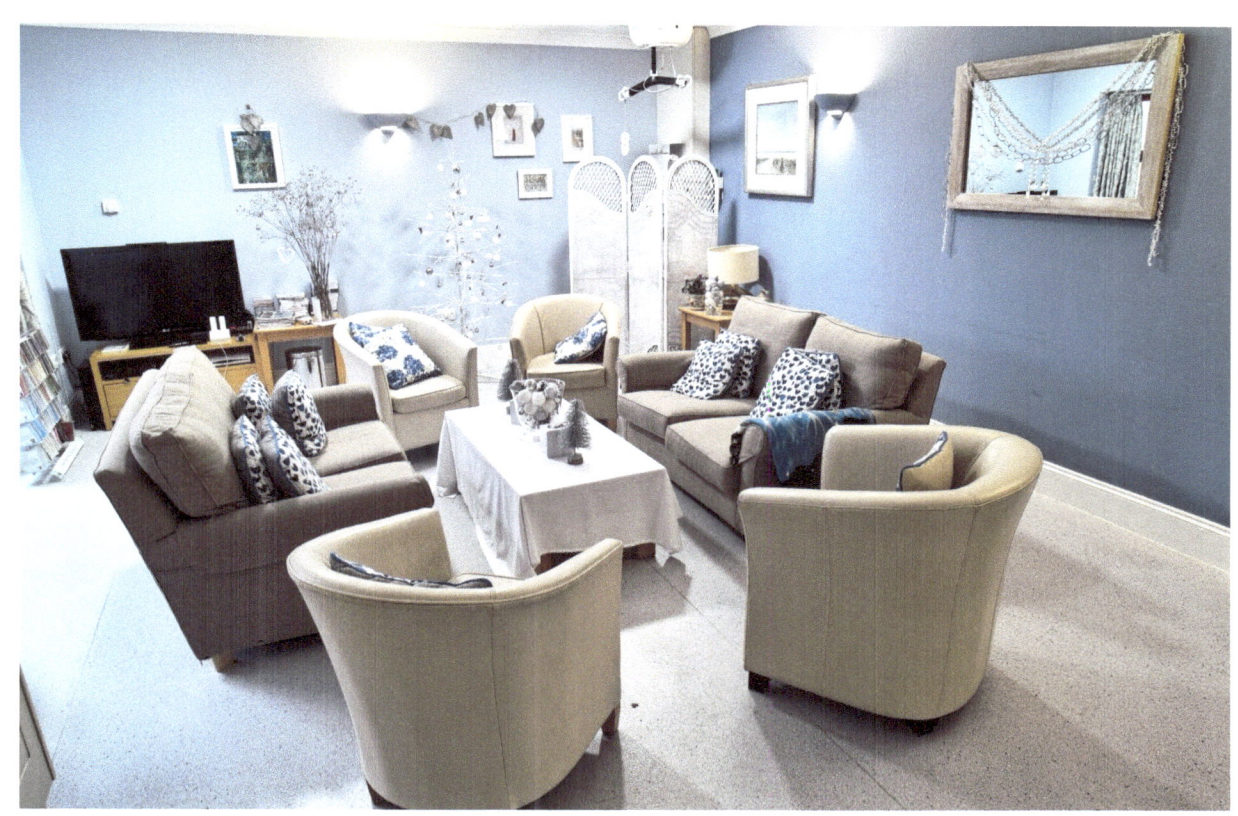

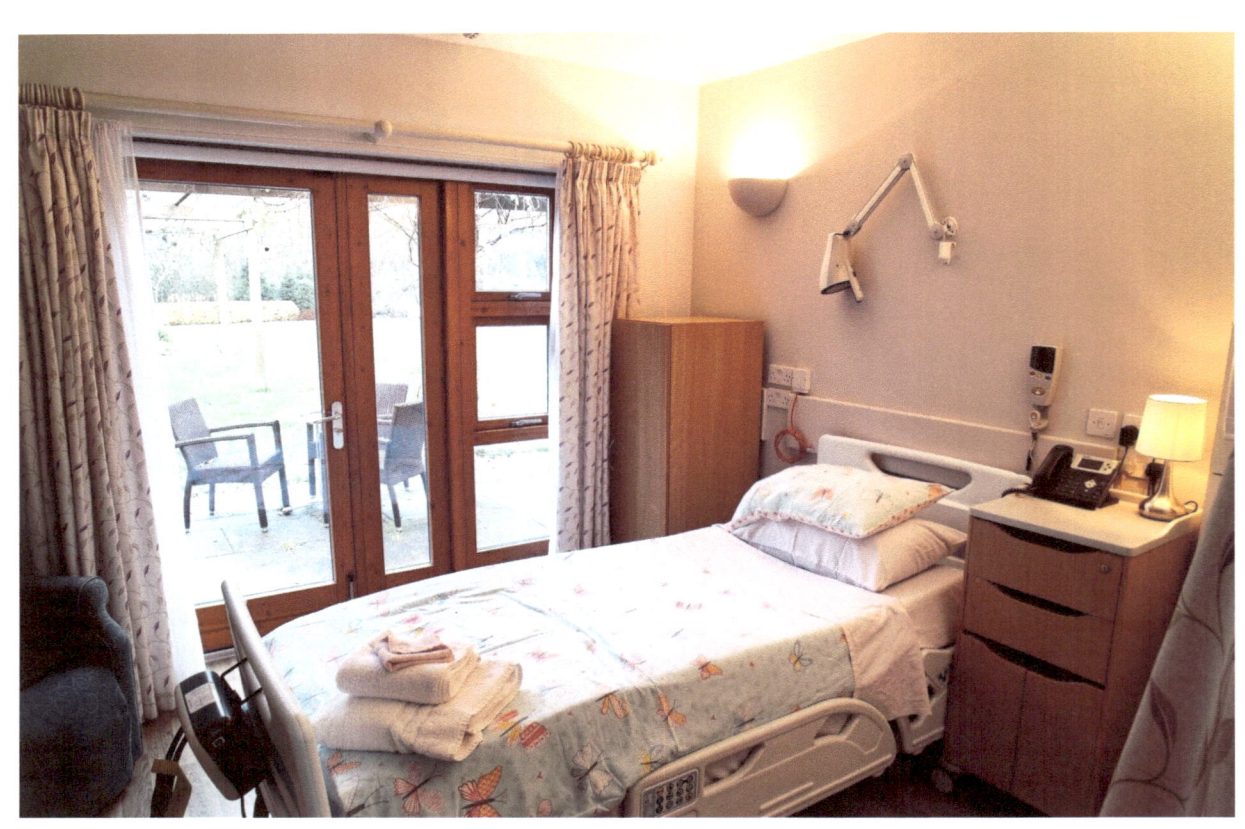

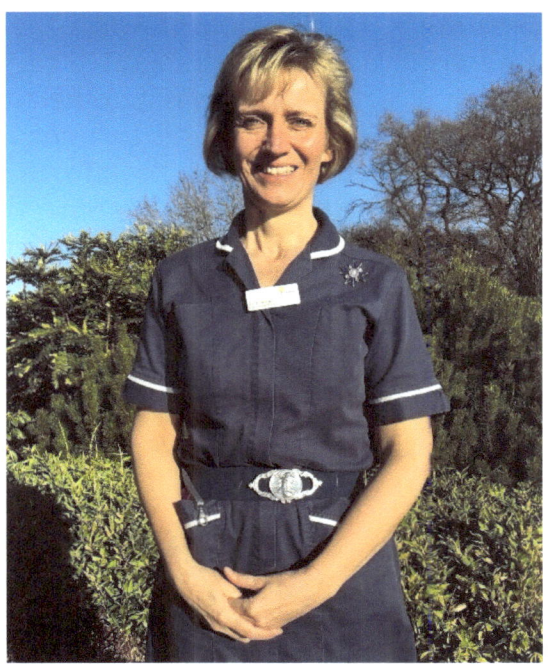

Jo
Practice Development Nurse

"I've worked at the Hospice since 2002, and I divide my time between the education department and the Inpatient Unit. I'm utterly passionate about my work and I still feel the same sense of privilege at working here as I did when I first joined. The values and desire to affect a positive influence on people's lives are part of who I am. The most satisfying part of my job is being by the bedside with patients and their loved ones - it's the place where my fondest and happiest, yet also my most emotionally charged and saddest memories are made. It's undeniably hard sometimes: I've had countless difficult conversations with people, yet just as many inspiring ones. To have the opportunity to hear people's stories is such a privilege and to work in an organisation that never thinks 'there's nothing more we can do' is amazing. Because there's always something we can do - even if we can't take away the sometimes painful reality of all of our mortality."

While so much good happens at the Hospice and through the teams in the community, another way in which the philosophy of holistic, integrated care can be shared is through the Hospice's thriving Education Programme. Training others to take the high standards of care back to their own workplaces, whether that is to a hospital, care home or another place altogether, is a key way of disseminating and reinforcing the ideals and practices that are central to The Hospice of St Francis. Combine that with offering clinical placements for those training to become the nurses and physicians of the future, and you can see that the reach of the Hospice is far wider than its four walls - or even the boundaries of its catchment area.

"Currently I am studying in my first year of sixth form and I aspire to study medicine at university in the future and hopefully become an oncologist. I began volunteering in the Inpatient Unit last summer in order to experience first-hand what it would be like to work in a medical environment, which is a very rare opportunity for someone of my age. Volunteering at the Hospice gave me the chance to meet and speak with patients, visitors and nurses, which has greatly improved my communication skills and taught me how to speak with compassion and confidence around a diverse range of people. I am very grateful to be part of the volunteering team at the Hospice as it truly is an extremely rewarding way to gain experience. Since I began volunteering, my passion to pursue a career in medical care has heightened as I have seen first-hand the impact that hospices, doctors and volunteers can have on the patients and it makes me extremely proud to be part of the team."

Rimsha, volunteer

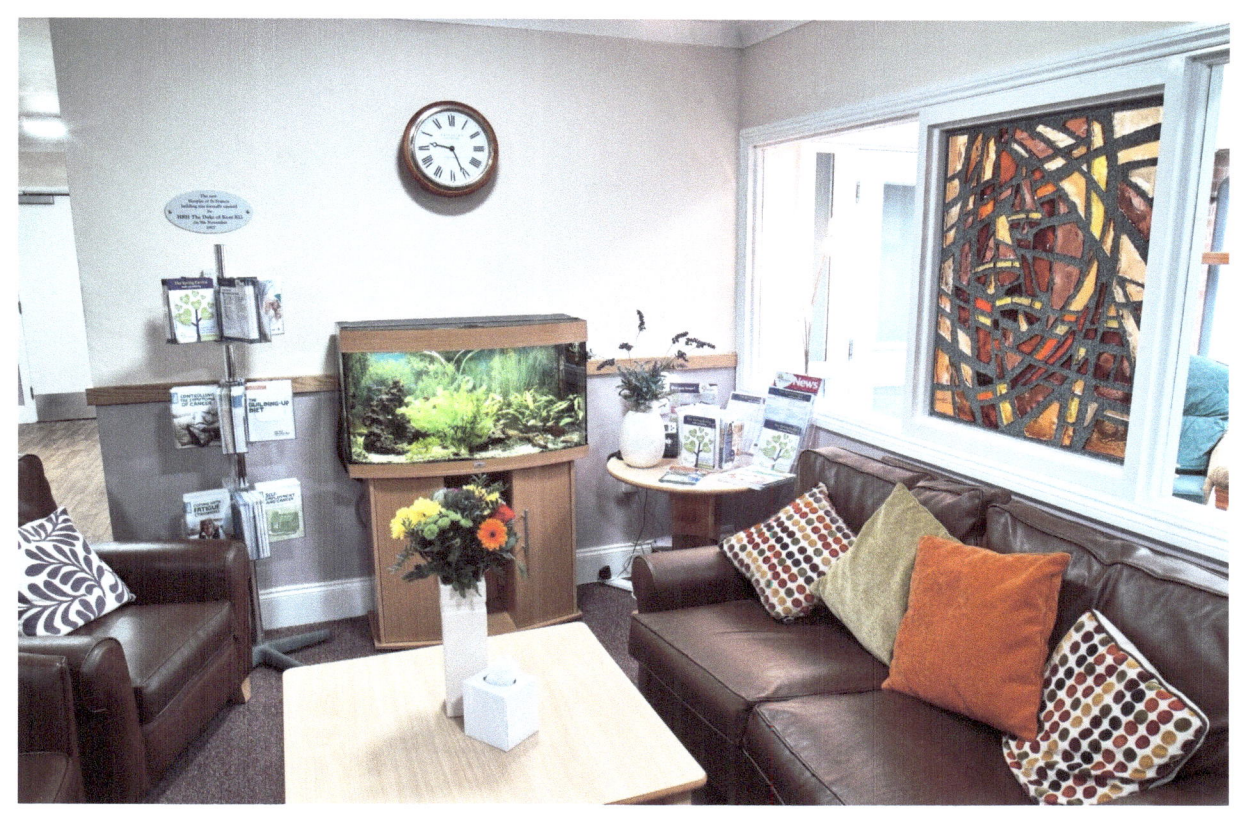

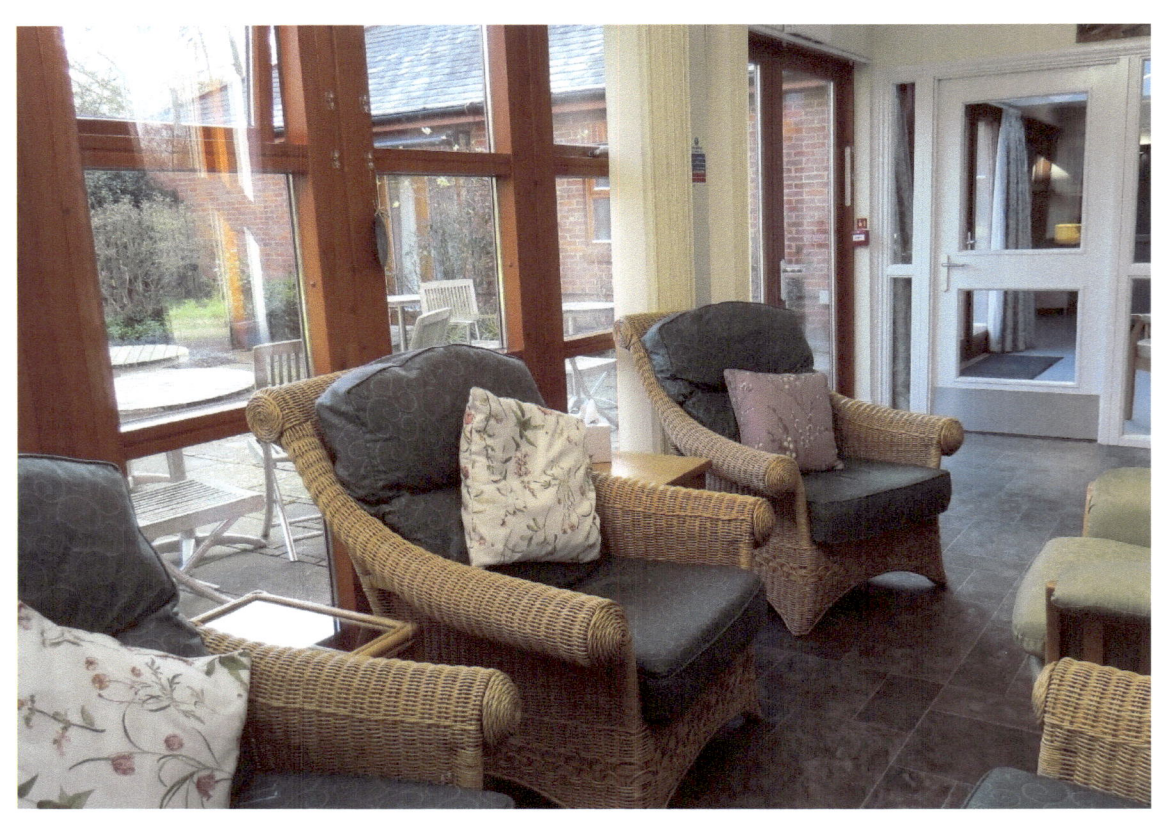

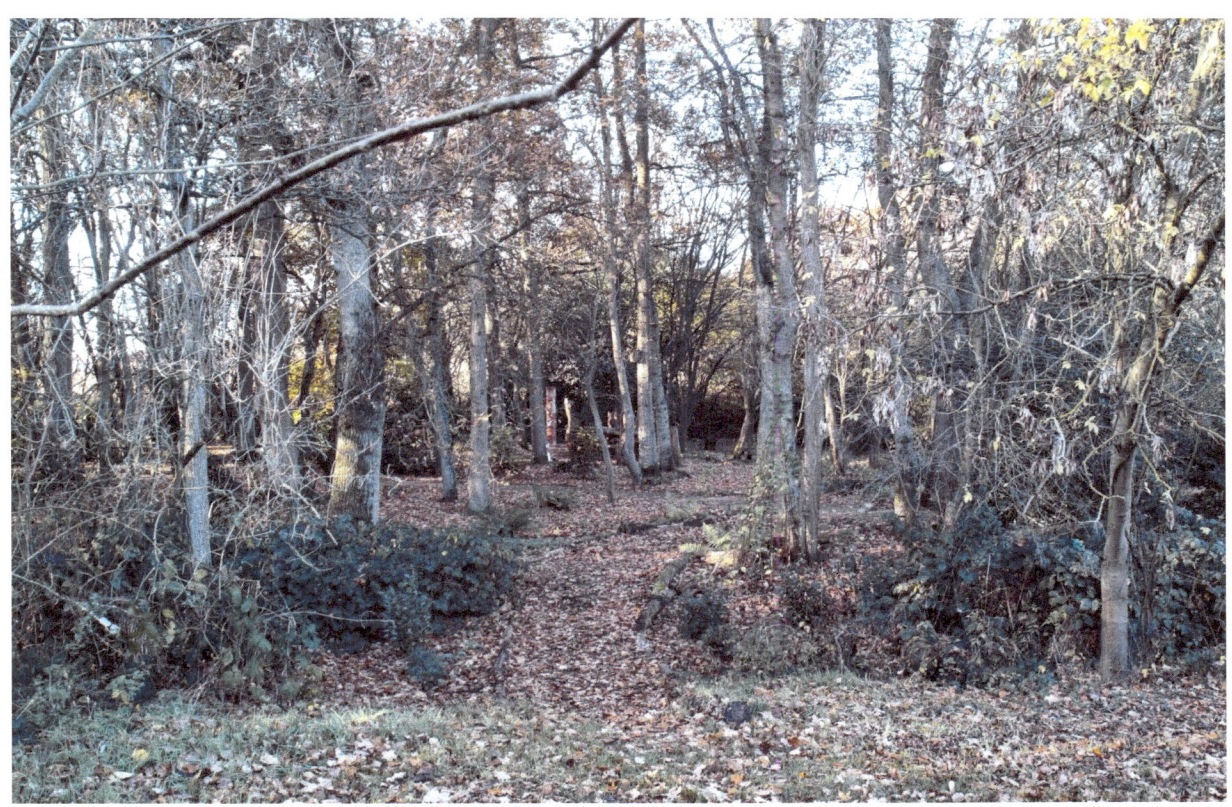

The woodland path is full of mystery and delightful surprises as one wanders slowly along. It is also very peaceful. A pile of logs will provide refuge for many tiny creatures who live among the leaf litter. Even in decay, nature creates new life. There are so many interesting little areas within the woodland trail, always inviting you to explore a little further while you take the air as the sun casts its benevolent light across the ground and points the way towards adventure - or towards the picnic table nestled among the trees. A mysterious path along the woodland trail looks very inviting, leading away from where the main Hospice buildings are situated. What lies ahead?

"When you are dependent for everything on another person, possibly in pain, unable to cope alone and focusing on the unknown, a single partner or care home assistant is not always enough. The busyness of a general hospital cannot always provide the calmness and emotional support that is needed. My father, lost in his own thoughts and frustrated by what remained of his life, was rescued by The Hospice of St Francis. Supported, nurtured, eased, calmed and cared for to the inevitable end in the right gentle environment by people who understood and had the time and the skills he needed."

David, family member

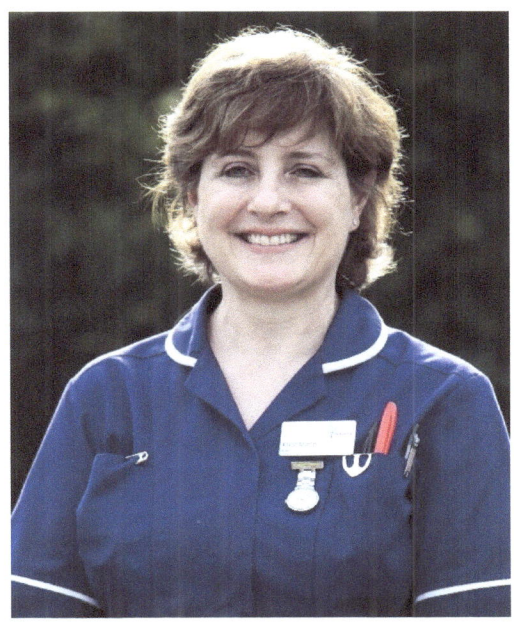

Karen
Sister and IPU Referrals Coordinator

"I have always wanted to be a nurse and whilst training, recognised that I wanted to care for patients who have cancer and so I trained to be an oncology nurse. As a student, I also explored the important work of Cicely Saunders, who said, 'You matter because you are you, and you matter to the end of your life.' Her words and work inspired me to pursue not only cancer nursing, and I have now been working as a palliative care nurse for more than seven years at The Hospice of St Francis. I learn from patients daily and marvel at their stoic tenacity and humour. Along with the rest of the team, I endeavour to ensure our patients live well and maintain laughter in their hearts. I feel honoured to play a small part in our patients' journey and offer support in any way, and I have always felt privileged to be part of such an inspired organisation, caring for people with life-limiting illnesses to try and help them facilitate their own dreams."

In the Inpatient Unit, the professionalism of the best in contemporary healthcare is brought together with the comfort of home. Every aspect of the IPU, as it is known, is focused on the safety, dignity and privacy of the patients cared for there - as well as for the families who sit with them. Many patients spend just a few days in the IPU, returning home having had difficult symptoms eased and brought under control, and some spend their final days in the quiet, compassionate care of the staff there. Each of the rooms opens out onto the Hospice gardens, filling the rooms with sunshine and the beauty of nature.

"I honestly can't praise the Hospice enough. They were just amazing. I lived there for a month at Maggie's side and there's not a single thing you could improve. The Hospice has many excellent facilities, including Jacuzzi baths, complementary therapies and beautiful grounds. All the staff were so very kind to us as a family."

Yogi, family member

"I was delighted with the range of services the Hospice could offer me, which were really tailored to me as an individual and are what makes the Hospice so special. The difference they have made to my life has been huge."

Amanda, patient

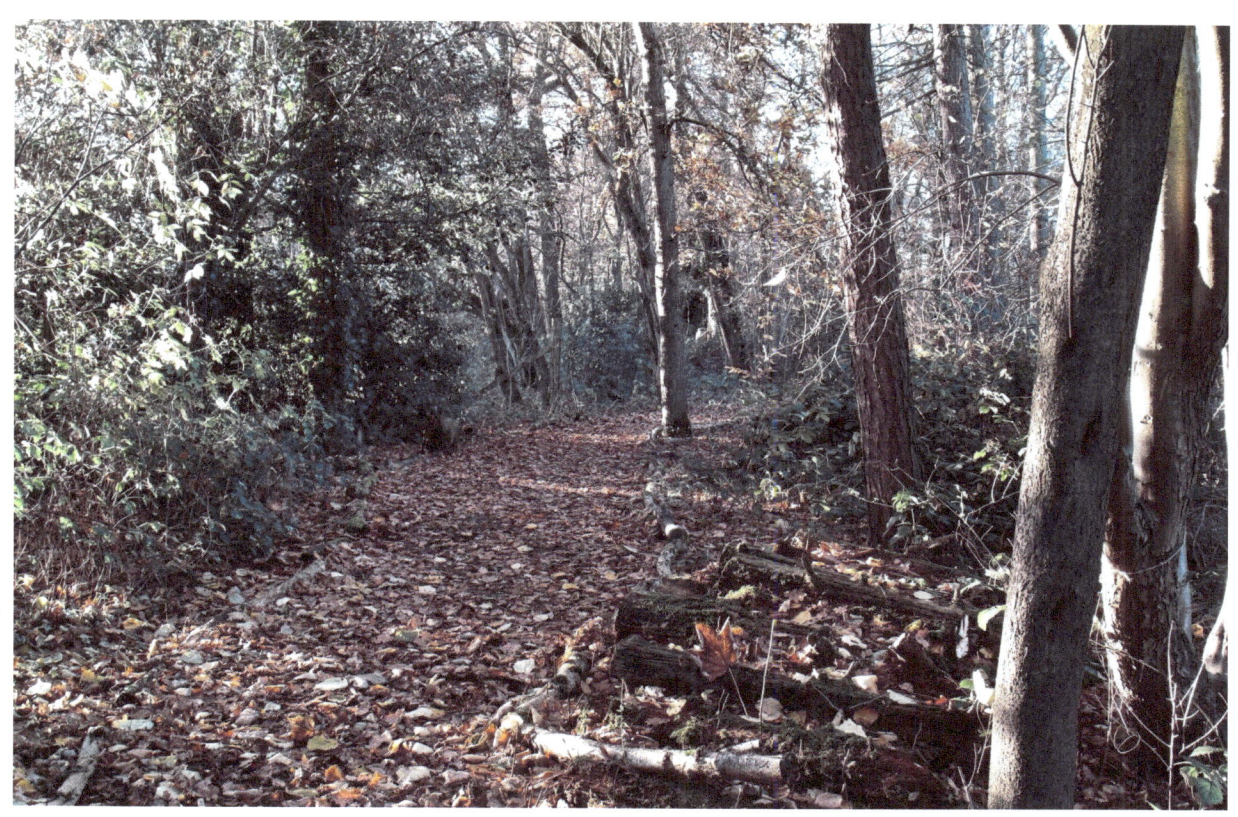

I do hope that you have enjoyed getting to know The Hospice of St Francis, and the individuals who make it so special, through the pages of this book. While it may be true that every hospice plays an important part in society, The Hospice of St Francis is exceptional - truly exceptional - and it is so through the expertise, unstinting effort and kindness of those you have met in this book, plus many others who serve as volunteers or who support the Hospice in so many other ways.

One might expect that a hospice would provide clinical expertise and support, but this is only a part of the story where The Hospice of St Francis is concerned. There is more. It is not just the support, but the way in which it is provided, with humanity and care for the individual, which defines all that is special about The Hospice of St Francis. The reassuring effect of this kindness upon the comfort and wellbeing of the patient is incalculable. Especially at a time which, for many, will be the most difficult period of their lives. Furthermore, this care and understanding does not stop with the patient, but extends to the family as well. In addition, The Hospice of St Francis nurses are very active within the community, liaising with outpatients, GPs, consultants, district nurses, hospitals and care homes, to ensure that patients are properly supported. Indeed, once taken under the wing of the Hospice, one has the feeling of being part of a large and loving family. It is a good feeling.

However, all of this wonderful care and attention does not occur automatically. It requires very careful planning and administration. In addition, it requires considerable funding. It may come as a surprise to some that the vast majority of funding for the Hospice comes from charitable donations, with only a very small amount (20%) being granted as official support from the Government. This funding must be renewed every year, year upon year. So please, please, do whatever you can to support this wonderful institution, whether by direct donation, volunteering or by other means. The Hospice of St Francis is a cornerstone of our town. Long may it prevail.

Julian Ashbourn

A Special Place

There is a place within my heart
Where very few may go
The door is opened late at night
When all is still, although

Sometimes a gentle voice is heard
Whispering through the haze
Of bustling times, wherein its words
Caress the careless days

Reminding me of what is true
Among all that I have seen
The world that's come within my view
In my time that has been

So fleeting here on this good Earth
With all its wonders dear
Of all that's not yet come to birth
While yet the night draws near

And now I may add to my store
Of precious memories there
The Hospice of St Francis
And all the loving care

That is brought to those who find
Their paths converging close
As if directed by a sign
Of that which matters most

And now the new day's rising sun
Warms me to the start
Of another chapter just begun
In that place within my heart

Julian Ashbourn

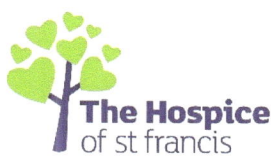

Registered Charity Number: 280825

The Hospice of St Francis
Spring Garden Lane
Off Shootersway
Northchurch
Berkhamsted
Hertfordshire
HP4 3GW

Tel: 01442 869550
Email: info@stfrancis.org.uk
Facebook: www.Facebook.com/TheHospiceofStFrancis
Twitter: @hospicstfrancis

www.ingramcontent.com/pod-product-compliance
Lightning Source LLC
Chambersburg PA
CBHW051021180526
45172CB00002B/425